Blueprints

PSYCHIATRY

FOURTH EDITION

Blueprints

PSYCHIATRY

FOURTH EDITION

Michael J. Murphy, MD, MPH
Instructor in Psychiatry
Harvard Medical School
Boston, Massachusetts
Assistant Psychiatrist
McLean Hospital
Belmont, Massachusetts

Ronald L. Cowan, MD, PhD
Assistant Professor of Psychiatry
Assistant Professor of Radiology and Radiological Sciences
Vanderbilt University Medical Center
Nashville, Tennessee

With the assistance of

David F. Street, MD
Psychiatry Resident Physician
Department of Psychiatry
Vanderbilt University
Nashville, Tennessee

Faculty Advisor

Lloyd I. Sederer, MD
Executive Deputy Commissioner for Mental Hygiene
Department of Health and Mental Hygiene
The City of New York
New York, New York

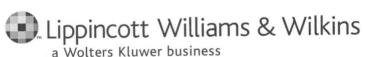
Lippincott Williams & Wilkins
a Wolters Kluwer business
Philadelphia • Baltimore • New York • London
Buenos Aires • Hong Kong • Sydney • Tokyo

Acquisitions Editor: Nancy Anastasi Duffy
Managing Editor: Kelly Horvath
Marketing Manager: Jennifer Kuklinski
Associate Production Manager: Kevin P. Johnson
Creative Director: Doug Smock
Compositor: International Typesetting and Composition
Printer: Quebecor World Dubuque

First Edition, Blackwell 1997
Second Edition, Blackwell 2001
Third Edition, Blackwell 2004

Library of Congress Cataloging-in-Publication Data

Murphy, Michael J.
  Blueprints Psychiatry / Michael J. Murphy, Ronald L. Cowan, Katie S. Fine—4th ed.
    p. ; cm.—(Blueprints)
  Includes index.
  ISBN 1-4051-0502-X
  1. Psychiatry—Outlines, syllabi, etc. I. Fine, Katie S. (Katie Snead) II. Title. III. Series.
  [DNLM: 1. Psychiatry—Examination Questions. WS 18.2 M339b 2007]
RJ48.3.M37 2007
618.92'00076—dc22   2006004933

Preface

*B*lueprints Psychiatry was conceived by a group of recent medical school graduates who saw a need for a thorough yet compact review of psychiatry that would adequately prepare students for the USMLE yet would be digestible in small pieces that busy residents can read during rare moments of calm between busy hospital and clinical responsibilities. Many students have reported that the book is also useful for the successful completion of the core and advanced psychiatry clerkships. We believe that the book provides a good overview of the field that the student should supplement with more in-depth reading. Before *Blueprints*, we felt that review books were either too cursory to be adequate or too detailed in their coverage for busy readers with little free time. We have kept the content current by repeated updates and revisions of the book while retaining a balance between comprehensiveness and brevity. Many changes have been made in response to user feedback. The structure of the book mirrors the major concepts and therapeutics of modern psychiatric practice. We cover each major diagnostic category, each major class of somatic and psychotherapeutic treatment, legal issues, and special situations that are unique to the field. We recommend that those preparing for USMLE read the book in chapter order but cross-reference when helpful between diagnostic and treatment chapters. We hope that *Blueprints Psychiatry* fits as neatly into your study regimen as it fits into your backpack or briefcase. You never know when you'll have a free moment to review for the boards!

Michael J. Murphy, MD, MPH

Acknowledgments

We acknowledge the faculty, staff, and trainees of the McLean Hospital, Harvard Medical School, and the Vanderbilt University Medical Center for their ongoing inspiration.

Ronald L. Cowan, MD, PhD
Michael J. Murphy, MD, MPH

Contents

Abbreviations

AA	Alcoholics Anonymous		IM	Intramuscular
ABG	Arterial blood gas		IPT	Intrapersonal therapy
ACLS	Advanced cardiac life support		IQ	Intelligence quotient
ACTH	Adrenocorticotropic hormone		IV	Intravenous
ADHD	Attention-deficit/hyperactivity disorder		LP	Lumbar puncture
AIDS	Acquired immunodeficiency syndrome		LSD	Lysergic acid diethylamine
ASP	Antisocial personality disorder		MAOI	Monoamine oxidase inhibitor
BAL	Blood alcohol level		MCV	Mean corpuscular volume
BID	Twice daily		MDMA	Ecstasy
cAMP	Adenosine monophosphate		MeCP2	Methyl-CpG-binding protein 2
CBC	Complete blood count		MR	Mental retardation
CBT	Cognitive-behavioral therapy		MRI	Magnetic resonance imaging
CNS	Central nervous system		NDRIs	Norepinephrine-dopamine reuptake inhibitors
CO_2	Carbon dioxide		NIDA	National Institute on Drug Abuse
CPR	Cardiopulmonary resuscitation		NMDA	*N*-Methyl-D-aspartate
CSF	Cerebrospinal fluid		NMS	Neuroleptic malignant syndrome
CT	Computerized tomography		NREM	Non-rapid eye movement
CVA	Cerebrovascular accident		OCD	Obsessive–compulsive disorder
DBT	Dialectical behavioral therapy		PCA	Patient-controlled analgesia
DID	Dissociative identity disorder		PCP	Phencyclidine
DSM-IV	*Diagnostic and Statistical Manual of Mental Disorders,* 4th edition		PMN	Polymorphonuclear leukocytes
			PO	By mouth
DT	Delirium tremens		PTSD	Posttraumatic stress disorder
ECG	Electrocardiogram		QD	Each day
ECT	Electroconvulsive therapy		REM	Rapid eye movement
EEG	Electroencephalogram		SES	Socioeconomic status
ED	Emergency department		SIADH	Syndrome of inappropriate antidiuretic hormone secretion
EPS	Extrapyramidal symptoms		SNRIs	Serotonin-noradrenergic reuptake inhibitors
EW	Emergency ward			
FBI	Federal Bureau of Investigation		SSRI	Selective serotonin-reuptake inhibitor
FDA	U.S. Food and Drug Administration		T_3	Tri-iodo thyronine
5HIAA	5-hydroxy indoleacetic acid		T_4	Tetra-iodo thyronine
5HT	5-hydroxy tryptamine		TCA	Tricyclic antidepressant
GABA	Gamma-amino butyric acid		TD	Tardive dyskinesia
GAD	Generalized anxiety disorder		TID	Three times daily
GHB	Gamma-hydroxybutyrate		TSH	Thyroid-stimulating hormone
GI	Gastrointestinal		VNS	Vagus nerve stimulation
HPF	High power field		WBC	White blood cell count
HIV	Human immunodeficiency virus		WISC-R	Wechsler Intelligence Scale for Children–Revised
ICU	Intensive care unit			

Psychotic Disorders

Psychotic disorders are a collection of disorders in which **psychosis**, defined as a gross impairment in reality testing, predominates the symptom complex. Specific psychotic symptoms include delusions, hallucinations, ideas of reference, and disorders of thought. Table 1-1 lists the *Diagnostic and Statistical Manual of Mental Disorders*, 4th edition (DSM-IV) classification of the psychotic disorders.

It is important to understand that psychotic disorders are different from mood disorders with **psychotic features**. Patients can present with a severe episode of depression and have delusions or with a manic episode with delusions and hallucinations. These patients do not have a primary psychotic disorder; rather, their psychosis is secondary to a mood disorder.

The diagnoses described below are among the most severely disabling of mental disorders. Disability is due in part to the extreme degree of social and occupational dysfunction associated with these disorders.

SCHIZOPHRENIA

Schizophrenia is a disorder in which patients have psychotic symptoms and social or occupational dysfunction that persists for at least 6 months.

EPIDEMIOLOGY

Schizophrenia affects 1% of the population. The typical age of onset is the early 20s for men and the late 20s for women. Women are more likely to have a "first break" later in life; in fact, about one third of women have an onset of illness after age 30. Schizophrenia is diagnosed disproportionately among the lower socioeconomic classes; although theories exist for this finding, none has been substantiated.

RISK FACTORS

Risk factors for schizophrenia include genetic risk factors (family history), prenatal and perinatal factors such as difficulties or infections during maternal pregnancy or delivery, neurocognitive abnormalities such as low premorbid intelligence quotient (IQ) or early childhood neurodevelopmental difficulties, urban living, migration to a different culture, and cannabis use (especially in susceptible individuals).

ETIOLOGY

The etiology of schizophrenia is unknown. There is a clear inheritable component, but familial incidence is sporadic and schizophrenia does occur in families with no history of the disease. Schizophrenia is widely believed to be a neurodevelopmental disorder. The most notable theory is the **dopamine hypothesis**, which posits that schizophrenia is due to hyperactivity in brain dopaminergic pathways. This theory is consistent with the efficacy of antipsychotics (which block dopamine receptors) and the ability of drugs (such as cocaine or amphetamines) that stimulate dopaminergic activity to induce psychosis. Postmortem studies also have shown higher numbers of dopamine receptors in specific subcortical nuclei of those with schizophrenia than in those with normal brains. More recent studies have focused on structural and functional abnormalities through brain imaging of patients with schizophrenia and control populations. No one finding or theory to date suffices to explain the etiology and pathogenesis of this complex

■ TABLE 1-1 Psychotic Disorders	
Schizophrenia	Brief psychotic disorder
Schizophreniform disorder	Shared psychotic disorder
Schizoaffective disorder	Delusional disorder

disease. Additional neurotransmitter systems, such as gamma-amino butyric acid (GABA) and glutamate and their neurons, are also implicated in the pathogenesis of schizophrenia.

CLINICAL MANIFESTATIONS

History and Mental Status Examination

Schizophrenia is a disorder characterized by symptoms that have been termed **positive** and **negative symptoms**, by a pattern of **social and occupational deterioration**, and by persistence of the illness for at least **6 months**. Positive symptoms are characterized by the **presence** of unusual thoughts, perceptions, and behaviors (e.g., hallucinations, delusions, agitation); negative symptoms are characterized by the **absence** of normal social and mental functions (e.g., lack of motivation, isolation, anergia, and poor self-care). The positive versus negative distinction was made in a nosologic attempt to identify subtypes of schizophrenia, as well as because some medications seem to be more effective in treating negative symptoms. Clinically, patients often exhibit both positive and negative symptoms at the same time. Table 1-2 lists common positive and negative symptoms.

To make the diagnosis, two (or more) of the following criteria must be met: hallucinations, delusions, disorganized speech, grossly disorganized or catatonic (mute or posturing) behavior, or negative symptoms. There must also be social or occupational dysfunction. The patient must be ill for at least 6 months.

Patients with schizophrenia generally have a history of abnormal premorbid functioning. The prodrome of schizophrenia includes poor social skills, social withdrawal, and unusual (although not frankly delusional) thinking. Inquiring about the premorbid history may help to distinguish schizophrenia from a psychotic illness secondary to mania or drug ingestion.

Patients with schizophrenia are at high risk for suicide. Approximately one third will attempt suicide

■ TABLE 1-2 Positive and Negative Symptoms of Schizophrenia	
Negative symptoms	
Affective flattening	Decreased expression of emotion, such as lack of expressive gestures
Alogia	Literally "lack of words," including poverty of speech and of speech content in response to a question
Asociality	Few friends, activities, interests; impaired intimacy, little sexual interest
Positive symptoms	
Hallucinations	Auditory, visual, tactile, or olfactory hallucinations; voices that are commenting
Delusions	Often described by content; persecutory, grandiose, paranoid, religious; ideas of reference, thought broadcasting, thought insertion, thought withdrawal
Bizarre behavior	Aggressive/agitated, odd clothing or appearance, odd social behavior, repetitive-stereotyped behavior

Adapted from Andreasen NC, Black DW, *Introductory textbook of psychiatry.* 3rd ed. Washington, DC: American Psychiatric Publishing, 2001.

and 10% will complete suicide. Risk factors for suicide include male gender, age <30 years, chronic course, prior depression, and recent hospital discharge.

DSM-IV recognizes five subtypes of schizophrenia: paranoid, disorganized, catatonic, undifferentiated, and residual. The subtypes of schizophrenia are useful as descriptors but have not been shown to be reliable or valid. Table 1-3 describes these subtypes.

Diagnostic Evaluation

The diagnostic evaluation for schizophrenia involves a detailed history, physical, and laboratory examination, preferably including brain magnetic resonance imaging (MRI). Medical causes, such as neuroendocrine abnormalities, psychostimulant abuse or dependence, and such brain insults as tumors or infection, should be ruled out.

■ TABLE 1-3 Subtypes of Schizophrenia	
Paranoid	Paranoid delusions, frequent auditory hallucinations, affect *not* flat
Catatonic	Motoric immobility or excessive, purposeless motor activity, maintenance of a rigid posture, echolalia
Disorganized	Disorganized speech, disorganized behavior, flat or inappropriate affect; not catatonic
Undifferentiated (probably most common)	Delusions, hallucinations, disorganized speech, catatonic behavior, negative symptoms; *criteria not met for paranoid, catatonic, or disorganized*
Residual	Met criteria for schizophrenia, now resolved, i.e., no hallucinations, no prominent delusions, etc., but *residual* negative symptoms or attenuated delusions, hallucinations, or thought disorder

Adapted from Andreasen NC, Black DW, *Introductory textbook of psychiatry*. 3rd ed. Washington, DC: American Psychiatric Publishing, 2001.

Differential Diagnosis

The differential diagnosis of an acute psychotic episode is broad and challenging (Table 1-4). Once a medical or substance-related condition has been ruled out, the task is to differentiate schizophrenia from a schizoaffective disorder, a mood disorder with psychotic features, a delusional disorder, or a personality disorder.

MANAGEMENT

Antipsychotic agents (also called neuroleptics) are primarily used in treatment. These medications are used to treat acute psychotic episodes and to maintain patients in remission or with chronic illness. Antipsychotic medications are discussed in Chapter 11. Combinations of several classes of medications are often prescribed in severe or refractory cases. **Psychosocial treatments**, including stable reality-oriented psychotherapy, family support, psycho-education, social and vocational skills training, and attention to details of living situation (housing, roommates, daily activities), are critical to the long-term management of

■ TABLE 1-4 Causes of Acute Psychotic Syndromes

Major psychiatric disorders
  Acute exacerbation of schizophrenia
  Atypical psychoses (e.g., schizophreniform)
  Depression with psychotic features
  Mania
Drug abuse and withdrawal
  Alcohol withdrawal
  Amphetamines and cocaine
  Phencyclidine (PCP) and hallucinogens
  Sedative-hypnotic withdrawal
Prescription drugs
  Anticholinergic agents
  Digitalis toxicity
  Glucocorticoids and adrenocorticotropic hormone (ACTH)
  Isoniazid
  L-Dopa and other dopamine agonists
  Nonsteroidal anti-inflammatory agents
  Withdrawal from monoamine oxidase inhibitors (MAOIs)
Other toxic agents
  Carbon disulfide
  Heavy metals
Neurologic causes
  AIDS encephalopathy
  Brain tumor
  Complex partial seizures
  Early Alzheimer's or Pick's disease
  Huntington's disease
  Hypoxic encephalopathy
  Infectious viral encephalitis
  Lupus cerebritis
  Neurosyphilis
  Stroke
  Wilson's disease
Metabolic causes
  Acute intermittent porphyria
  Cushing's syndrome

(Continued)

■ TABLE 1-4 Causes of Acute Psychotic Syndromes (*continued*)

Early hepatic encephalopathy

Hypo- and hypercalcemia

Hypoglycemia

Hypo- and hyperthyroidism

Paraneoplastic syndromes (limbic encephalitis)

Nutritional causes

   Niacin deficiency (pellagra)

   Thiamine deficiency (Wernicke–Korsakoff syndrome)

   Vitamin B_{12} deficiency

From Rosenbaum JF, Arana GW, Hyman SE, et al. *Handbook of psychiatric drug therapy.* 5th ed. Philadelphia: Lippincott Williams & Wilkins, 2005.

these patients. Complications of schizophrenia include those related to antipsychotic medications, secondary consequences of poor health care and impaired ability to care for oneself, and increased rates of suicide. Once diagnosed, schizophrenia is a chronic remitting/relapsing disorder with impaired interepisode function. Poorer prognosis occurs with early onset, a history of head trauma, or comorbid substance abuse.

🔑 1-1 KEY POINTS

1. Schizophrenia is characterized by psychosis and social/occupational dysfunction.
2. Symptoms must last for at least 6 months.
3. Schizophrenia has a 10% suicide rate (approximately one third attempt).
4. Treatment is with antipsychotics and psychosocial support.

SCHIZOAFFECTIVE DISORDER

Patients with schizoaffective disorder have psychotic episodes that **resemble schizophrenia but with prominent mood disturbances**. Their psychotic symptoms, however, must persist for some time in the absence of any mood syndrome.

EPIDEMIOLOGY

Lifetime prevalence is estimated at 0.5% to 0.8%. Age of onset is similar to schizophrenia (late teens to early 20s).

RISK FACTORS

Risk factors for schizoaffective disorder are not well established but likely overlap with those of schizophrenia and affective disorders.

ETIOLOGY

The etiology of schizoaffective disorder is unknown. It may be a variant of schizophrenia, a variant of a mood disorder, a distinct psychotic syndrome, or simply superimposed mood disorder and psychotic disorder.

CLINICAL MANIFESTATIONS

History and Mental Status Examination

Patients with schizoaffective disorder have the typical symptoms of schizophrenia and coincidentally a major mood disturbance, such as a manic or depressive episode. They must also have periods of illness in which they have psychotic symptoms **without a major mood disturbance**. Mood disturbances need to be present for a substantial portion of the illness.

There are two subtypes of schizoaffective disorder recognized in the DSM-IV, **depressive** and **bipolar**, which are determined by the nature of the mood-disturbance episodes.

Diagnostic Evaluation

The diagnostic evaluation for schizoaffective disorder is similar to other psychiatric conditions and involves a detailed history, physical, and laboratory examination, preferably including brain magnetic resonance imaging (MRI). Medical conditions producing secondary behavioral symptoms should be ruled out.

Differential Diagnosis

Mood disorders with psychotic features, as in mania or psychotic depression, are different from schizoaffective disorder in that patients with schizoaffective disorder have persistence (for at least 2 weeks) of the psychotic symptoms after the mood symptoms have resolved. Schizophrenia is differentiated from schizoaffective disorder by the absence of a prominent mood disorder in the course of the illness.

It is important to distinguish the prominent negative symptoms of the patient with schizophrenia from the **lack of energy** or **anhedonia** in the depressed patient with schizoaffective disorder. More distinct symptoms of a mood disturbance (such as depressed mood and sleep disturbance) should indicate a true coincident mood disturbance.

MANAGEMENT

Patients are treated with medications that target the psychosis and the mood disorder. Typically, these patients require the **combination of an antipsychotic medication and a mood stabilizer**. Mood stabilizers are described in Chapter 13. An antidepressant or electroconvulsive therapy may be needed for an acute depressive episode. Psychosocial treatments are similar for schizoaffective disorder and schizophrenia. Complications of schizoaffective disorder include those related to antipsychotic and mood stabilizer medications, secondary consequences of poor health care and impaired ability to care for oneself, and increased rates of suicide. Prognosis is better than for schizophrenia and worse than for bipolar disorder or major depression. Patients with schizoaffective disorder are more likely than those with schizophrenia but less likely than mood-disordered patients to have a remission after treatment.

🔑 1-2 KEY POINTS

1. In schizoaffective disorder, there are mood disturbances *with* psychotic episodes and there are periods of psychosis *without* a mood disturbance.
2. Treatment is with antipsychotics and mood stabilizers.
3. The prognosis for schizoaffective disorder is better than for schizophrenia but worse than for a mood disorder.

SCHIZOPHRENIFORM DISORDER

Essentially, schizophreniform disorder is schizophrenia that fails to last for 6 months and does not involve social withdrawal.

EPIDEMIOLOGY

The validity of this diagnosis is under question. Outcome studies of this disorder indicate that most patients may go on to develop full-blown schizophrenia, whereas others appear to develop a mood disorder. The diagnosis of schizophreniform disorder may, however, help to avoid premature diagnosis of patients with schizophrenia before some other disorder, such as bipolar disorder, manifests itself.

RISK FACTORS

Because most patients with schizophreniform disorder are eventually diagnosed with schizophrenia, risk factors are likely similar for the two groups.

ETIOLOGY

At this time, the etiology is unknown. At least one study found similarities in brain structure abnormalities between patients with schizophrenia and those with schizophreniform disorder.

CLINICAL MANIFESTATIONS

History and Mental Status Examination

Schizophreniform disorder is essentially **short-course schizophrenia** without the requirement of social withdrawal. Patients with this disorder have what appears to be a "full-blown" episode of schizophrenia, including delusions, hallucinations, disorganized speech, or negative symptoms, but the duration of illness including prodromal, active, and residual phases, is from 1 to 6 months. The diagnosis changes to schizophrenia once the symptoms have extended past 6 months, even if only residual symptoms are left.

Differential Diagnosis

Care must be taken to distinguish schizophreniform disorder from a manic or depressive episode with psychotic features. Other causes of an acute psychosis must be ruled out (substance-induced or due to a general medical condition).

MANAGEMENT

The disorder is by definition **self-limited**. When symptoms cause severe impairment, treatment is similar to that for the acute treatment of psychosis in schizophrenia.

1-3 KEY POINTS

1. Schizophreniform disorder resembles schizophrenia.
2. The disorder resolves completely in less than 6 months.
3. Either schizophrenia or bipolar disorder most often results.
4. The disorder is self-limited.

DELUSIONAL DISORDER

Delusional disorder is characterized by nonbizarre delusions without other psychotic symptoms. It is rare, its course is chronic, and treatment is supportive.

EPIDEMIOLOGY

This disorder is rare, with a prevalence of <0.05%. Generally, onset is in middle to late life; it affects women more often than men. Its course is generally **chronic** with remission uncommon.

ETIOLOGY

The etiology is unknown. Often, psychosocial stressors appear to be etiologic, for example, following **migration**. In migration psychosis, the recently immigrated person develops persecutory delusions. Many patients with delusional disorder have a paranoid character premorbidly. Paranoid personality disorder has been found in families of patients with delusional disorder.

CLINICAL MANIFESTATIONS

History and Mental Status Examination

This disorder is characterized by well-systematized **nonbizarre delusions** about things that could happen in real life (such as being followed, poisoned, infected, loved at a distance, having a disease, being deceived by one's spouse or significant other). The delusions must be present for at least 1 month. Other than the delusion, the patient's social adjustment may be normal.

The patient must not meet criteria for schizophrenia. Any mood disorder must be brief relative to the

TABLE 1-5 Delusional Disorder Subtypes

Erotomanic	A person becomes falsely convinced that another person is in love with him or her.
Grandiose	A person becomes falsely convinced that he or she has special abilities or is in other ways much more important than reality indicates.
Jealous	A person becomes falsely convinced that his or her lover is unfaithful.
Persecutory	A person becomes falsely convinced that others are out to harm him or her and that he or she is being conspired against in general.
Somatic	A person becomes falsely convinced that he or she has a bodily function disorder, for example, organ dysfunction, body odor, or parasite infection.
Mixed	A person is so diagnosed when no single delusional theme predominates.
Unspecified	A person is so diagnosed when a single delusional theme cannot be determined or when the predominant delusional theme does not match subtype criteria

duration of the illness. The DSM-IV recognizes seven subtypes of delusional disorder (Table 1-5).

DIFFERENTIAL DIAGNOSIS

It is important to rule out other psychiatric or medical illnesses that could have caused the delusions. Thereafter, delusional disorder must be distinguished from major depression with psychotic features, mania, schizophrenia, and paranoid personality.

MANAGEMENT

Trials of antipsychotics are appropriate but are often ineffective. The primary treatment is **psychotherapy**, taking care neither to support nor to refute the delusion but to maintain an **alliance** with the patient. Without such an alliance, most patients fall out of treatment; with an alliance, over time, the patient may relinquish the delusions.

BRIEF PSYCHOTIC DISORDER

In brief psychotic disorder, the patient experiences a full psychotic episode that is **short-lived**. It can be temporally related to some stressor or occur postpartum, but is also seen **without any apparent antecedent**.

EPIDEMIOLOGY

There is insufficient data available to determine prevalence and sex ratio.

ETIOLOGY

Etiology is unknown. However, the disorder seems to be associated with borderline personality disorder and schizotypal personality disorder.

CLINICAL MANIFESTATIONS

History and Mental Status Examination

In brief psychotic disorder, the patient develops psychotic symptoms that last for at least 1 day but no more than 1 month, followed by eventual return to premorbid functioning. Patients can exhibit any combination of delusions, hallucinations, disorganized speech, or grossly disorganized behavior. There are three recognized subtypes: **with marked stressors** (formerly known as brief reactive psychosis), **without marked stressors**, and **postpartum**. Patients with the postpartum subtype typically develop symptoms within 1 to 2 weeks after delivery that resolve within 2 to 3 months.

Differential Diagnosis

It is important to rule out schizophrenia, especially if the disorder worsens or persists for more than a month (except for postpartum psychosis, which may last 2 to 3 months). A mood disorder such as mania or depression with psychotic features must be ruled out.

MANAGEMENT

Hospitalization may be necessary to protect the patient. Treatment with antipsychotics is common, although the condition is by definition self-limited and no specific treatment is required. The containing environment of the hospital milieu may be sufficient to help the patient recover.

References

Freedman R. Schizophrenia. *N Engl J Med*. 2003 Oct 30;349(18):1738–1749. Review.

Maki P, Veijola J, Jones PB, et al. Predictors of schizophrenia—a review. *Br Med Bull*. 2005 Jun 9;73–74:1–15.

Winterer G, Weinberger DR. Genes, dopamine and cortical signal-to-noise ratio in schizophrenia. *Trends Neurosci*. 2004 Nov;27(11):683–690. Review.

Chapter 2

Mood Disorders

Mood disorders are among the most common diagnoses in psychiatry. Mood is a persistent emotional state (as differentiated from affect, which is the external display of feelings). There are three major categories of mood disorders according to the *Diagnostic and Statistical Manual of Mental Disorders*, 4th edition: unipolar mood disorders (major depressive disorder, dysthymic disorder), bipolar mood disorders (bipolar I disorder, bipolar II disorder, and cyclothymic disorder), and mood disorders having a known etiology (substance-induced mood disorder and mood disorder due to a general medical condition) (Table 2-1).

The best available evidence suggests that mood disorders lie on a continuum with normal mood. Although mania and depression are often viewed as opposite ends of the mood spectrum, they can occur simultaneously in a single individual within a brief period, giving rise to the concept of mixed mood states.

UNIPOLAR DISORDERS

Unipolar disorders are major depressive disorder and dysthymic disorder.

MAJOR DEPRESSIVE DISORDER

Major depressive disorder is diagnosed after a single episode of major depression (Table 2-2). It is characterized by emotional changes, primarily depressed mood, and by so-called vegetative changes, consisting of alterations in sleep, appetite, and energy levels. A major depressive episode can occur at any time from early childhood to old age.

Epidemiology

The lifetime prevalence (will occur at some point in a person's life) rate for major depressive disorder is 5% to 20%. The female–male ratio is 2:1. Race distributions appear equal, and socioeconomic variables do not seem to be a factor. The incidence (rate of new cases) is greatest between the ages of 20 and 40 and decreases after the age of 65. Approximately 2.5% of children and 8% of adolescents suffer from depression; depression affects 1% to 3% of elderly persons.

Etiology

Psychological theories of depression generally view interpersonal losses (actual or perceived) as risk factors for developing depression. In fact, available evidence suggests that childhood loss of a parent or loss of a spouse is associated with depression. Classic psychoanalytic theories center on ambivalence toward the lost object (person), although more recent theories focus on the critical importance of the object relationship in maintaining psychic equilibrium and self-regard. The cognitive-behavioral model views cognitive distortions as the primary events that foster a negative misperception of the world, which in turn generate negative emotions. The learned helplessness model (based on animal studies) suggests that depression arises when individuals come to believe they have no control over the stresses and pains that beset them.

Biologic, familial, and genetic data support the idea of a biologic diathesis in the genesis of depression. Genetic studies show that depression is found to be concordant more often in monozygotic twins than in dizygotic twins. Unipolar depression in a parent leads to an increased incidence of both unipolar and bipolar mood disorders in their offspring.

Neurotransmitter evidence points to abnormalities in amine neurotransmitters as mediators of depressive states: The evidence is strongest for deficiencies in norepinephrine and serotonin.

9

■ TABLE 2-1 Classification of Mood Disorder

Unipolar	Bipolar	Etiologic
Major depressive disorder	Bipolar I disorder	Substance-induced mood disorder
Dysthymic disorder	Bipolar II disorder	Mood disorder due to general medical condition
	Cyclothymic disorder	

Neuroendocrine abnormalities in the hypothalamic–pituitary–adrenal axis are often present in depression and suggest a neuroendocrine link.

Sleep disturbances are nearly universal complaints in depressed persons. Objective evidence from sleep studies reveals that deep sleep (delta sleep, stages 3 and 4) is decreased in depression and that rapid-eye-movement (REM) sleep alterations include increased time spent in REM and earlier onset of REM in the sleep cycle (decreased latency to REM).

Clinical Manifestations

History and Mental Status Examination

A major depressive disorder is diagnosed if a patient experiences at least one episode of major depression and does not meet criteria for bipolar disorder or etiologic mood disorder. Major depression is characterized by emotional and vegetative changes. Emotional changes most commonly include depressed mood with feelings of sadness, hopelessness, guilt, and despair. Irritability may be the primary mood complaint in some cases. Vegetative symptoms include alterations in sleep, appetite, energy, and libido. In addition to the symptoms seen in adults, children present with school avoidance, problems with authority, frequent headaches or stomachaches, and anger outbursts. Elderly persons, often beset by grief, loss, or medical illness, present with the usual adult symptoms and with higher rates of co-occurring anxiety.

Major depression is frequently **recurrent**. The usual duration of an untreated episode (Fig. 2-1A) is 6 to 12 months. Of patients diagnosed with major depression, 15% die by suicide at some point in their lifetime. White men over age 65 have a suicide rate that is five times that of the general population.

■ TABLE 2-2 Criteria for Major Depressive Episode

Mood: depressed mood most of the day, nearly every day

Sleep: insomnia or hypersomnia

Interest: marked decrease in interest and pleasure in most activities

Guilt: feelings of worthlessness or inappropriate guilt

Energy: fatigue or low energy nearly everyday

Concentration: decreased concentration or increased indecisiveness

Appetite: increased or decreased appetite or weight gain or loss

Psychomotor: psychomotor agitation or retardation

Suicidality: recurrent thoughts of death, suicidal ideation, suicidal plan, suicide attempt

General criteria for a major depressive episode require five or more of the above symptoms to be present for at least 2 weeks; one symptom must be *depressed mood* or *loss of interest* or *pleasure*. These symptoms must be a change from prior functioning and cannot be due to a medical condition, cannot be substance-induced, and cannot be due to bereavement. The symptoms must also cause *distress* or *impairment*.

From American Psychiatric Association, *Diagnostic and statistical manual of mental disorders*, 4th ed, text rev. Washington, DC: American Psychiatric Association, 2000.

Differential Diagnosis

Mood disorders secondary to (induced by) medical illnesses or substance abuse are the primary differential diagnoses. Psychotic depression must be differentiated from schizophrenia; negative symptoms of schizophrenia can mimic depression. Persons with major depression may eventually meet criteria for bipolar disorder.

Management

Depression is responsive to **psychotherapy** and **pharmacotherapy**. Milder cases may be treated with brief psychotherapy interventions alone. For more severe cases, antidepressant medications combined with psychotherapy are superior to medications or psychotherapy alone. Among the psychotherapies, supportive, cognitive-behavioral, and brief interpersonal therapies have the most data to support their efficacy.

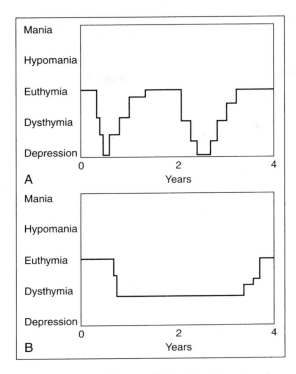

Figure 2-1 • Unipolar mood disorders. **A:** major depressive disorder; **B:** dysthymic disorder.

There is a long tradition of psychodynamic psychotherapy in treating depression, although it has not been well studied empirically.

There are many classes of antidepressants available that are effective and are usually chosen according to side-effect profiles. At present, available classes of antidepressants include tricyclic antidepressants, selective serotonin reuptake inhibitors, monoamine oxidase inhibitors, and atypical antidepressants. In addition, lithium, thyroid hormone, and psychostimulants may be used as augmentative treatments.

Children and adolescents with depression benefit from some antidepressants and from psychotherapy as well. They may be at higher risk of suicide during active pharmacologic treatment and sufferers should be carefully followed by a mental health specialist. Elderly persons with depression do best when low dosages of antidepressants are initiated and raised slowly in conjunction with psychotherapy.

Electroconvulsive therapy (ECT) is used in psychotic, severe, or treatment-refractory depressions or when medications are contraindicated (e.g., in elderly or debilitated individuals). Vagal nerve stimulation, a novel bio-electrical treatment involving the electrical

stimulation of the vagus nerve via a surgically implanted device has shown some promise as a potential treatment for major depression, although current use is still limited by cost and availability. Antipsychotic medications are an essential adjunct to antidepressants in psychotic depressions and may be helpful even in nonpsychotic depression. Anxiolytics may be used as adjuncts to antidepressants in depression with high levels of anxiety, although more-sedating antidepressants may suffice. Phototherapy can be used for seasonal mood disorders.

🔑 2-1 KEY POINTS

1. Major depression is a unipolar mood disorder.
2. The condition affects people of all ages and is often recurrent.
3. Major depression has a 15% suicide rate.
4. Combined psychotherapy and pharmacotherapy is the best treatment for all ages.

DYSTHYMIC DISORDER

Dysthymic disorder is a mild, chronic form of major depression.

Epidemiology

The lifetime prevalence is 6%.

Etiology

Because dysthymia is often conceptualized as a milder, chronic form of major depression, similar etiologies are generally attributed to dysthymia.

Clinical Manifestations

History and Mental Status Examination

Dysthymic disorder is a chronic and less severe form of major depression. The diagnosis of dysthymia requires that an individual experience a minimum of 2 years of chronically depressed mood most of the time (Fig. 2-1B). Associated symptoms and complaints may include change in appetite and sleep, fatigue, decreased concentration, and hopelessness. Dysthymia can be chronic and difficult to treat. At times, major depressive episodes may co-occur, giving rise to the term double depression.

Differential Diagnosis

Major depression and etiologic mood disorders are the primary differential diagnostic considerations.

Management

Treatment is similar to major depression except that psychotherapy may play a larger role and the course of treatment may be more protracted.

⚷ 2-2 KEY POINTS

1. Dysthymia is a unipolar mood disorder.
2. The condition is chronic, lasting at least 2 years.
3. Dysthymia is often refractory to treatment.

BIPOLAR DISORDERS

The bipolar disorders are bipolar I disorder, bipolar II disorder, and cyclothymia.

BIPOLAR I DISORDER

Bipolar I disorder is the most serious of the bipolar disorders and is diagnosed after at least one episode of mania (Table 2-3). Patients with bipolar I disorder typically also experience major depressive episodes in the course of their lives.

Epidemiology

The lifetime prevalence is 0.4% to 1.6% and the male–female ratio is equal. There are no racial variations in incidence.

Etiology

Genetic and familial studies reveal that bipolar I disorder is associated with increased bipolar I, bipolar II, and major depressive disorders in first-degree relatives. X linkage has been demonstrated in some studies but remains controversial. Mania can be precipitated by psychosocial stressors, and there is evidence that sleep/wake cycle perturbations may predispose a person to mania.

Clinical Manifestations

History and Mental Status Examination

Bipolar I disorder is defined by the occurrence of mania (or a mixed episode). A single manic episode

■ TABLE 2-3 Criteria for Manic Episode
Three to four of the following criteria are required during the elevated mood period:
Self-esteem: highly inflated, grandiosity
Sleep: decreased need for sleep, rested after only a few hours
Speech: pressured
Thoughts: racing thoughts and flight of ideas
Attention: easy distractibility
Activity: increased goal-directed activity
Hedonism: high excess involvement in pleasurable activities (sex, spending, travel)
General criteria for a manic episode require a clear period of persistently *elevated, expansive, or irritable mood* lasting 1 week or severe enough to require hospitalization. These symptoms must be a change from prior functioning and cannot be due to a medical condition and cannot be substance-induced. The symptoms also must cause distress or impairment.

From American Psychiatric Association, *Diagnostic and statistical manual of mental disorders*, 4th ed, text rev. Washington, DC: American Psychiatric Association, 2000.

is sufficient to meet diagnostic requirements; most patients, however, have recurrent episodes of mania typically intermixed with depressive episodes. The criteria for a manic episode are outlined in Table 2-3.

The first episode of mania usually occurs in the early 20s. Manic episodes are typically briefer than depressive episodes. The transition between mania and depression occurs without an intervening period of euthymia in about two of three patients (Fig. 2-2A). Lifetime suicide rates range from 10% to 15%.

Children can present with bipolar disorder that resembles the adult-type but differs according to age and developmental level. Very young children might present with uncontrollable giggling, slightly older children might try to teach their grammar school class in the presence of their teacher, adolescents might present with severe anger outbursts and agitation. Co-occurring psychiatric problems and psychosocial difficulties are the norm. Most children with bipolar disorder have more than one relative with the condition. A first episode of bipolar disorder

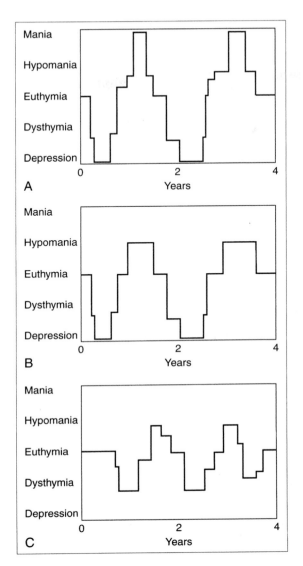

Figure 2-2 • Bipolar mood disorders. **A:** bipolar I disorder; **B:** bipolar II disorder; **C:** cyclothymic disorder.

in elderly individuals is rare. Medical or neurological causes of new bipolar disorder in an older person should be thoroughly investigated.

Differential Diagnosis

Mania may be induced by antidepressant treatment, including antidepressant medications, psychostimulants, ECT, and phototherapy. When this occurs, the patient is diagnosed with substance-induced mood disorder, not bipolar disorder. Mood disorder due to a general medical condition is the other major differential consideration. Schizoaffective disorder, borderline

personality disorder, and depression with agitation are also considerations.

Management

Persons experiencing a manic episode often have poor insight and resist treatment. Pharmacologic interventions for acute mania include **antipsychotics** in conjunction with **benzodiazepines** (for rapid tranquilization) and initiation of **mood stabilizer** medication. Antipsychotics are frequently used in mania with and without psychotic features. Lithium is the most commonly used mood stabilizer, but valproic acid is quite effective and is more effective for the rapid-cycling variant of mania. Carbamazepine, lamotrigine, gabapentin, and long-acting benzodiazepines are used if first-line treatments fail. Some atypical antipsychotics, particularly clozapine, quetiapine, olanzapine, and aripiprazole, appear to act as mood stabilizers and are increasingly being used for maintenance of bipolar disorder. ECT for mania, mixed episodes, or depressed episodes is used in patients with medication intolerance and where a more immediate response is medically or psychiatrically needed (e.g., to treat a severely suicidal patient). Combination medication therapy is more common than monotherapy, although studies on the safety and effectiveness of such combinations are lacking. Children and adolescents are treated with medications similar to those of adults, often in combination, but with even fewer studies backing up various treatment strategies.

Mood stabilizer maintenance therapy is essential in preventing the recurrence of mania and appears to decrease the recurrence of depression. Psychotherapy is used to encourage medication compliance, to help patients come to terms with their illness, and to help repair some of the interpersonal damage done while ill (e.g., infidelity, hostility, squandering money). Care must be taken when prescribing antidepressants for depression or dysthymia because of their role in prompting more severe or more frequent manic episodes.

🔑 2-3 KEY POINTS

1. Bipolar I disorder is a biphasic mood disorder affecting adults as well as children.
2. The disorder is cyclic.
3. The suicide rate is 10% to 15%.
4. Maintenance treatment with mood stabilizers is required; combination therapy is common.

BIPOLAR II DISORDER

Bipolar II disorder is similar to bipolar I disorder except that mania is absent in bipolar II disorder and **hypomania** (a milder form of elevated mood than mania) is the essential diagnostic finding.

Epidemiology

Lifetime prevalence is about 0.5%. Bipolar II disorder may be more common in women.

Etiology

Current evidence implicates the same factors as for bipolar I.

Clinical Manifestations

History and Mental Status Examination

Bipolar II disorder is characterized by the occurrence of hypomania and episodes of major depression in an individual who has never met criteria for mania or a mixed state. Hypomania is determined by the same symptom complex as mania, but the symptoms are less severe, cause less impairment, and usually do not require hospitalization. Bipolar II disorder is **cyclic;** the course of untreated bipolar II is presented in Figure 2-2B. Suicide occurs in 10% to 15%.

Differential Diagnosis

Same as for bipolar I disorder.

Management

Treatment is the same as for bipolar I disorder, although hypomanic episodes typically do not require as aggressive a treatment regimen as does mania. Care must be taken in prescribing antidepressants for depression or dysthymia because of their role in prompting more severe or frequent hypomanic episodes.

🔑 2-4 KEY POINTS

1. Bipolar II disorder is a biphasic mood disorder with hypomania.
2. The disorder is recurrent.
3. The suicide rate is 10% to 15%.

CYCLOTHYMIC DISORDER

Cyclothymic disorder is a recurrent, chronic, mild form of bipolar disorder in which mood typically oscillates between hypomania and dysthymia. It is not diagnosed if a person has experienced either a manic episode or a major depressive episode.

Epidemiology

The lifetime prevalence of cyclothymic disorder is 0.4% to 1%. The rate appears equal in men and women, although women more often seek treatment.

Etiology

Familial and genetic studies reveal an association with other mood disorders.

Clinical Manifestations

History and Mental Status Examination

Cyclothymic disorder is a milder form of bipolar disorder consisting of **recurrent mood disturbances** between hypomania and dysthymic mood. A single episode of hypomania is sufficient to diagnose cyclothymic disorder; however, most individuals also have dysthymic periods. Cyclothymic disorder is never diagnosed when there is a history of mania or major depressive episode or mixed episode. The course of untreated cyclothymic disorder is depicted in Figure 2-2C.

Differential Diagnosis

The principal differential is among other unipolar and bipolar mood disorders, substance-induced mood disorder, and mood disorder due to a general medical condition. Personality disorders (especially border-line) with labile mood may be confused with cyclothymic disorder.

Management

Psychotherapy, mood stabilizers, and antidepressants are used. However, persons with cyclothymia may never seek medical attention for their mood symptoms.

🔑 2-5 KEY POINTS

1. Cyclothymic disorder is a biphasic mood disorder without frank mania or depression.
2. The disorder is chronic and recurrent.

MOOD DISORDERS WITH KNOWN ETIOLOGY

SUBSTANCE-INDUCED MOOD DISORDER

Substance-induced mood disorder is diagnosed when medications, other psychoactive substances, ECT, or phototherapy are proximate events and the likely cause of the mood disturbance. All the aforementioned types of mood disorder (e.g., unipolar, bipolar) may occur.

MOOD DISORDER DUE TO A GENERAL MEDICAL CONDITION

This category is for mood disturbances apparently caused by a medical illness. Endocrine disorders, such as thyroid and adrenal dysfunction, are common etiologies. Postpartum mood disorders are excluded from the criteria; they are modifiers of unipolar and bipolar mood disorders (see above).

SUBTYPES AND MODIFIERS

Various diagnostic specifiers can be applied to specific subtypes of mood disorders. These have prognostic and treatment implications and may prove to have etiologic implications.

Melancholic: Melancholic depression is a severe form of depression associated with guilt, remorse, loss of pleasure, and extreme vegetative symptoms.

Postpartum: Postpartum depression occurs within 4 weeks of delivery. The presence of one episode of postpartum mood disorder is strongly predictive of a recurrence.

Seasonal: Seasonal mood disorders show a consistent seasonal pattern of variation. The most common pattern is a worsening of depression during the fall and winter with improvement in the spring. The reverse is sometimes true. If the depression is a component of a bipolar disorder, the manic and hypomanic episodes may show a seasonal association.

Atypical: Atypical depressions show a pattern of hypersomnia, increased appetite or weight gain, mood reactivity, long-standing rejection sensitivity, anergia, and leaden paralysis.

Rapid Cycling: Patients with bipolar disorder may have frequent (rapid) cycles. To meet criteria for rapid cycling, four mood disturbances per year must be present. The suicide rate may be higher than in non-rapid cyclers.

Catatonic: The catatonic specifier is applied to mood disorders when there are pronounced movement abnormalities, including motoric immobility or excessive purposeless motor activity, maintenance of a rigid posture, mutism, stereotyped movement, echolalia (repetition of a word or phrase just spoken by another person), and echopraxia (repetition of movements made by another person).

References

American Psychiatric Association. Practice guideline for the treatment of patients with bipolar disorder (revision). *Am J Psychiatry.* 2002;159(4 Suppl): 1–50.

Rush AJ et al. Vagus nerve stimulation for treatment-resistant depression: a randomized, controlled acute phase trial. *Biol Psychiatry.* 2005 Sep 1;58(5):347–354.

Trivedi MH, Rush AJ, et al. Clinical results for patients with major depressive disorder in the Texas Medication Algorithm Project. *Arch Gen Psychiatry.* 2004 Jul;61(7):669–680.

Youngstrom EA, Findling RL, Youngstrom JK, et al. Toward an evidence-based assessment of pediatric bipolar disorder. *J Clin Child Adolesc Psychol.* 2005 Sep;34(3):433–448.

Anxiety Disorders

The term **anxiety** refers to many states in which the sufferer experiences a sense of impending threat or doom that is not well defined or realistically based. Anxiety can be adaptive or pathologic, transient or chronic, and has a variety of psychologic and physical manifestations. **Anxiety disorders** are a heterogeneous group of disorders in which the feeling of anxiety is the major element. They are the most prevalent group of psychiatric disorders; according to the Epidemiological Catchment Area study, 7.3% of all Americans meet the *Diagnostic and Statistical Manual of Mental Disorders*, 3rd edition (DSM-III; the DSM version used at the time) criteria at a given point in time (so-called point prevalence). Anxiety disorders listed in the *Diagnostic and Statistical Manual of Mental Disorders*, 4th edition (DSM-IV) are shown in Table 3-1.

PANIC DISORDER AND AGORAPHOBIA

Panic disorder is characterized by recurrent unexpected panic attacks that can occur *with or without* agoraphobia. Agoraphobia is a disabling condition in which patients fear places from which escape might be difficult. Whether occurring as distinct disorders or together, panic disorder and agoraphobia are common, sometimes disabling, conditions.

EPIDEMIOLOGY

Panic disorder occurs more frequently in women, with a lifetime prevalence of 2% to 3%. The typical onset is in the 20s, with most cases beginning before age 30.

Agoraphobia also occurs more frequently in women, with a lifetime prevalence of between 2% and 6%. Only one third of patients with agoraphobia also have panic disorder. However, most patients with agoraphobia seen clinically also have panic disorder. This apparent contradiction is due to the fact that patients with agoraphobia alone are unlikely to seek treatment.

ETIOLOGY

The etiology of panic disorder is unknown. There are several popular biologic theories involving carbon dioxide (CO_2) hypersensitivity (potentially involving medullary cholinergic function), abnormalities in lactate metabolism, an abnormality of the locus coeruleus (a region in the brain that regulates level of arousal), and elevated central nervous system catecholamine levels. The gamma-amino butyric acid (GABA) receptor also has been implicated as etiologic because patients respond well to benzodiazepines and because panic is induced in patients with anxiety disorders using GABA antagonists.

Theorists posit that panic attacks are a conditioned response to a fearful situation. For example, a person has an automobile accident and experiences severe anxiety, including palpitations. Thereafter, palpitations alone, experienced during exercise or any sympathetic nervous system response, may induce the conditioned response of a panic attack.

CLINICAL MANIFESTATIONS

History and Mental Status Examination

Panic disorder is characterized by **recurrent unexpected panic attacks** that can occur with or without agoraphobia (see below). Panic attacks typically come on

■ TABLE 3-1 Anxiety Disorders
Panic disorder *with agoraphobia*
Panic disorder *without agoraphobia*
Agoraphobia
Social phobia
Specific phobia
Obsessive–compulsive disorder
Generalized anxiety disorder
Acute stress disorder
Posttraumatic stress disorder
Substance-induced anxiety disorder
Anxiety disorder due to a general medical condition
Anxiety disorder not otherwise specified

■ TABLE 3-2 DSM-IV Criteria for Panic Attack
A discrete period of intense fear or discomfort, in which four (or more) of the following symptoms developed abruptly and reached a peak within 10 minutes:
• Palpitations, pounding heart, or accelerated heart rate
• Sweating
• Trembling or shaking
• Sensations of shortness of breath or smothering
• Feeling of choking
• Chest pain or discomfort
• Nausea or abdominal distress
• Feeling dizzy, unsteady, lightheaded, or faint
• Derealization (feelings of unreality) or depersonalization (being detached from oneself)
• Fear of losing control or going crazy
• Fear of dying
• Paresthesias
• Chills or hot flushes

Adapted from American Psychiatric Association, *Diagnostic and statistical manual of mental disorders*, 4th ed. Washington, DC: American Psychiatric Association, 2000.

suddenly, peak within minutes, and last 5 to 30 minutes. The patient must experience 4 of the 13 typical symptoms of panic outlined in Table 3-2.

To warrant the diagnosis, one of the following must occur for at least 1 month: persistent concern about having additional attacks, worry about the implications of the attack (losing control, "going crazy"), or a significant change of behavior related to the attacks (e.g., restriction of activities).

Agoraphobia is a disabling complication of panic disorder but can also occur in patients with no history of panic disorder. It is characterized by an **intense fear of places or situations** in which escape might be difficult (or embarrassing). Patients with agoraphobia and panic disorder typically fear having a panic attack in a public place and being embarrassed or unable to escape. Those with agoraphobia alone (two thirds of those with agoraphobia) simply avoid public arenas but do not have panic attacks. Although some patients with agoraphobia are so disabled that they are homebound, many are comforted by the presence of a companion, allowing them to enter some public places with less anxiety.

Diagnostic Evaluation

Panic disorder is diagnosed after taking a thorough history and performing necessary physical and laboratory examinations to rule out medical causes. In particular, cardiac conditions, such as rhythm disturbances, valvular abnormalities, and coronary artery disease, need to be carefully excluded. Use of psychostimulants such as cocaine or crystal methamphetamine must also be ruled out.

Differential Diagnosis

Panic attacks should be distinguished from the direct physiologic effects of a substance or a general medical condition (particularly cardiac conditions or partial complex epilepsy). The panic attacks also cannot be accounted for by another mental disorder, such as social phobia or obsessive–compulsive disorder (OCD).

MANAGEMENT

The main treatments for panic disorder are pharmacotherapy and cognitive-behavioral therapy or their combination. Specific **tricyclic antidepressants** (TCAs), specific **monoamine oxidase inhibitors** (MAOIs), **selective serotonin reuptake inhibitors** (SSRIs), and high-potency **benzodiazepines** have been shown to be effective in controlled studies. **Cognitive-behavioral** therapy (CBT) involves the use of relaxation exercises and desensitization combined with education aimed at helping patients to understand that their panic attacks are a result of misinterpreting bodily sensations. Patients can then learn that the sensations are innocuous and self-limited, which diminishes the panicky response. **Exposure therapy**, in which the patient incrementally confronts a feared stimulus, has been shown to be effective in treating agoraphobia.

3-1 KEY POINTS

1. Panic disorder is characterized by recurrent unexpected panic attacks.
2. Panic disorder can be seen with or without agoraphobia.
3. Panic disorder is treated with antidepressants and benzodiazepines and cognitive-behavioral techniques.
4. Agoraphobia is fear of not being able to (or being too embarrassed to) escape a place or situation.
5. Agoraphobia most often occurs alone (without panic).
6. Agoraphobia can be a complication of panic disorder.
7. Agoraphobia is treated with exposure therapy.

SPECIFIC PHOBIA

Specific phobia is an anxiety disorder characterized by intense fear of particular objects or situations (e.g., snakes, heights). It is the most common psychiatric disorder.

EPIDEMIOLOGY

Specific phobias are more prevalent in women than men and occur with a lifetime prevalence of 25%. Typical onset is in childhood, with most cases occurring before age 12.

ETIOLOGY

Phobic disorders, including specific phobia, tend to run in families. Behavioral theorists argue that phobias are learned by being paired with traumatic events.

CLINICAL MANIFESTATIONS

History and Mental Status Examination

A phobia is an irrational fear of a specific object, place, activity, or situation that is out of proportion to any actual danger. To meet the DSM-IV criteria for specific phobia, a patient must experience a marked, persistent fear that is recognized by the patient to be excessive or unreasonable and is cued by the presence or anticipation of a specific object or situation. In addition, exposure to the stimulus must almost invariably provoke the anxiety reaction, and the avoidance of or distress over the feared situation must impair everyday activities or relationships. For those younger than age 18, symptoms must persist for at least 6 months.

Differential Diagnosis

The principal differential diagnosis is another mental disorder (such as avoidance of school in separation anxiety disorder) presenting with anxiety or fearfulness.

MANAGEMENT

Specific childhood phobias tend to remit spontaneously with age. When they persist into adulthood, they often become chronic. However, they rarely cause disability. Exposure therapy in the form of **systematic desensitization** or **flooding** is the treatment of choice. There is little role for medication.

3-2 KEY POINTS

1. Specific phobia is an intense fear of a certain object, place, activity, or situation.
2. Specific phobia occurs in 25% of the population at some point in their lifetime, usually with onset before age 12.
3. Treatment is with systematic desensitization and flooding.

SOCIAL PHOBIA

Social phobia is an anxiety disorder in which patients have an intense fear of being scrutinized in social or public situations (e.g., giving a speech, speaking in class). The disorder may be **generalized** or **limited** to specific situations.

EPIDEMIOLOGY

Social phobias occur equally among men and women and affect 3% to 5% of the population. The typical onset is in adolescence, with most cases occurring before age 25.

ETIOLOGY

Phobic disorders, including social phobia, tend to run in families. Behavioral theorists argue that phobias are learned by being paired with traumatic events. Some theorists posit that hypersensitivity to rejection is a psychological antecedent of social phobia.

CLINICAL MANIFESTATIONS

History and Mental Status Examination

Social phobias are characterized by the fear of situations in which the person is exposed to unfamiliar people or to possible scrutiny by others. Exposure to the feared social situation must almost invariably provoke an anxiety reaction. Avoidance of or distress over the feared situation must impair everyday activities or relationships. For those younger than age 18, symptoms must persist for at least 6 months. Social phobia can either be generalized (the patient fears nearly all situations) or limited to specific situations.

Differential Diagnosis

The principal differential diagnosis is another mental disorder (such as avoidance of school in separation anxiety disorder) presenting with anxiety or fearfulness.

MANAGEMENT

Mild cases of social phobia can be treated with CBT, but many cases require medication. MAOIs, beta-blockers, SSRIs, alprazolam, and gabapentin have proved successful in treating social phobia. SSRIs appear to be the most effective pharmacotherapy. CBT uses the exposure therapy techniques of flooding and systematic desensitization to reduce anxiety in feared situations. Supportive individual and group psychotherapy is helpful to restore self-esteem and to encourage venturing into feared situations.

🔑 3-3 KEY POINTS

1. Social phobia is fear of exposure to scrutiny by others.
2. Social phobia has a lifetime prevalence of 3% to 5%, typically occurring before age 25.
3. The condition can be generalized or limited.
4. Treatment is with MAOIs, beta-blockers, SSRIs, alprazolam, or gabapentin and with CBT.

GENERALIZED ANXIETY DISORDER

Generalized anxiety disorder (GAD) is characterized by intense pervasive worry over virtually every aspect of life associated with **physical manifestations** of anxiety.

EPIDEMIOLOGY

The lifetime prevalence of GAD is approximately 5%. The typical age of onset is in the early 20s, but the disorder may begin at any age.

ETIOLOGY

Twin studies suggest that GAD has both inherited and environmental etiologies. Serotonergic, noradrenergic, and GABA-ergic neurotransmitter systems have been studied in relation to GAD, but the biologic etiology remains obscure. Cognitive-behavioral theorists posit that GAD is due to cognitive distortions in which patients misperceive situations as dangerous when they are not.

CLINICAL MANIFESTATIONS

History and Mental Status Examination

Patients with generalized anxiety disorder worry excessively about virtually every aspect of their lives (job performance, health, marital relations, and social life). They do not have panic attacks, phobias, obsessions, or compulsions; rather, they experience pervasive anxiety and worry (apprehensive expectation) about a number of events or activities that occur most days for at least 6 months. They must also have difficulty controlling the worry, and it must be associated with at least three of the following symptoms: restlessness, easily fatigued, difficulty concentrating or mind going blank, irritability, muscle tension, and sleep disturbance.

Differential Diagnosis

The focus of the anxiety and worry in GAD must not be symptomatic of another axis I disorder. For example, the anxiety and worry cannot be about having a panic attack (as in panic disorder) or being embarrassed in public (as in social phobia).

MANAGEMENT

The pharmacologic treatment of GAD is with **benzodiazepines, buspirone** (a non-benzodiazepine anxiolytic), **SSRIs, gabapentin,** or **beta-blockers**. Although benzodiazepines are very effective, the duration of treatment is limited by the risk of tolerance and dependence. **Relaxation techniques** are also used in treatment with some success.

🔑 3-4 KEY POINTS

1. GAD is intense worry over every aspect of life.
2. GAD is characterized by difficulty controlling the worry.
3. The disorder is associated with physical manifestations of anxiety.
4. Treatment is with benzodiazepines, buspirone, SSRIs, beta-blockers, gabapentin, and relaxation techniques.

POSTTRAUMATIC STRESS DISORDER

Posttraumatic stress disorder (PTSD) is an anxiety disorder characterized by the **persistent re-experience of a trauma, efforts to avoid recollecting the trauma,** and **hyperarousal** (Table 3-3).

EPIDEMIOLOGY

The prevalence of PTSD is estimated at 0.5% among men and 1.2% among women. PTSD may occur at any age from childhood through adulthood and may begin hours, days, or even years after the initial trauma.

■ TABLE 3-3 Posttraumatic Stress Disorder
Re-experience of the trauma
Efforts to avoid recollection of the trauma
Hyperarousal

ETIOLOGY

The central etiologic factor in PTSD is the trauma. There may be some necessary predisposition to PTSD because not all people who experience similar traumas develop the syndrome. Magnetic resonance imaging studies support a finding of altered hippocampal volume in PTSD.

CLINICAL MANIFESTATIONS

History and Mental Status Examination

People with PTSD have endured a traumatic event (e.g., combat, physical assault, rape, explosion) in which they experienced, witnessed, or were confronted with actual or potential death, serious physical injury, or a threat to physical integrity. The traumatic event is subsequently re-experienced through repetitive intrusive images or dreams or through recurrent illusions, hallucinations, or flashbacks of the event. In an adaptive attempt, these patients make efforts to avoid recollections of the event, often through psychological mechanisms (e.g., dissociation, numbing) or actual avoidance of circumstances that will evoke recall. They also experience feelings of detachment from others and exhibit evidence of autonomic hyperarousal (e.g., difficulty sleeping, exaggerated startle response).

Differential Diagnosis

Symptoms that resemble PTSD may be seen in depression, GAD, panic disorder, OCD, and dissociative disorder. When symptoms resemble PTSD, verify that there also are symptoms from all three categories; if not, consider one of the above diagnoses.

MANAGEMENT

Treatment is with a combination of **symptom-directed** psychopharmacologic agents and **psychotherapy** (individual or group). SSRIs used for at least 6 months appear to be the most effective treatment for reducing symptoms of PTSD. TCAs and MAOIs may also be effective. Propranolol and other beta-blockers may have a role in preventing the development of PTSD if given early after trauma. Psychotherapy is effective and is typically tailored to the nature of the trauma, degree of coping skills, and the support systems available to the patient.

🔑 3-5 KEY POINTS

1. PTSD occurs in response to trauma.
2. PTSD is characterized by re-experience of the trauma, efforts to avoid recalling the trauma, and hyperarousal.
3. Treatment is with medications directed at specific symptoms and with psychotherapy.

OBSESSIVE–COMPULSIVE DISORDER

OCD is an anxiety disorder in which patients experience recurrent obsessions and compulsions that cause significant distress and occupy a significant portion of their lives.

EPIDEMIOLOGY

The lifetime prevalence of OCD is 2% to 3%. Typical onset of the disorder is between the late teens and early 20s, but one third of patients show symptoms of OCD before age 15.

ETIOLOGY

Behavioral models of OCD claim that obsessions and compulsions are produced and sustained through classic and operant conditioning. Interestingly, OCD is seen more frequently after brain injury or disease (e.g., head trauma, seizure disorders, Huntington's disease), and twin studies show that monozygotic twins have a higher concordance rate than dizygotic twins; these findings support a biologic basis for the disorder. The neurotransmitter **serotonin** has been implicated as a mediator in obsessive thinking and compulsive behaviors. Neuroimaging evidence to date suggests that multiple brain regions are affected.

CLINICAL MANIFESTATIONS

History and Mental Status Examination

Patients with OCD experience obsessions and compulsions. **Obsessions** are recurrent intrusive ideas, thoughts, or images that cause significant anxiety and distress; **compulsions** are repetitive purposeful physical or mental actions that are generally performed in response to obsessions. The compulsive "rituals" are meant to neutralize the obsessions, diminish anxiety, or somehow magically prevent a dreaded event or situation.

Differential Diagnosis

It is important to distinguish the *obsessional* thinking of OCD from the *delusional* thinking of schizophrenia or other psychotic disorders. Obsessions are usually unwanted, resisted, and recognized by patients as coming from their own thoughts, whereas delusions are generally regarded as distinct from patients' thoughts and are typically not resisted.

MANAGEMENT

CBT, clomipramine, and SSRIs have been shown to be quite effective in treating OCD. Although poorly studied, the behavioral techniques of **systematic desensitization, flooding**, and **response prevention** have been used successfully to treat compulsive rituals. For example, someone who fears contamination from an object will hold the object repeatedly in therapy while simultaneously being prevented from carrying out the ritual associated with the dreaded object.

🔑 3-6 KEY POINTS

1. OCD is characterized by recurrent obsessions and compulsions.
2. OCD causes distress and wastes time by compelling patients to carry out various obsessions/compulsions/rituals.
3. Lifetime prevalence is 2% to 3%.
4. Treatment with CBT, clomipramine, and SSRIs, and with systematic desensitization, flooding, and response prevention.

References

Battaglia M, Ogliari A. Anxiety and panic: from human studies to animal research and back. *Neurosci Biobehav Rev.* 2005 Feb;29(1):169–179.

Kripke C. Is pharmacotherapy useful in social phobia? *Am Fam Physician.* 2005 May 1;71(9): 1700–1701.

Mataix-Cols D, Rosario-Campos MC, Leckman JF. A multidimensional model of obsessive-compulsive disorder. *Am J Psychiatry.* 2005 Feb;162(2): 228–238.

Mitte K, Noack P, Steil R, et al. A meta-analytic review of the efficacy of drug treatment in generalized anxiety disorder. *J Clin Psychopharmacol.* 2005 Apr;25(2):141–150.

Ursano RJ, Bell C, Eth S, et al, and Work Group on ASD and PTSD; Steering Committee on Practice Guidelines. Practice guideline for the treatment of patients with acute stress disorder and posttraumatic stress disorder. *Am J Psychiatry.* 2004 Nov;161 (11 Suppl):3–31.

Personality Disorders

Personality disorders are coded on Axis II in the *Diagnostic and Statistical Manual of Mental Disorders*, 4th edition (DSM-IV). Ten types of personality disorders are grouped into clusters based on similar overall characteristics. There are three recognized personality disorder clusters: **odd and eccentric, dramatic and emotional**, and **anxious and fearful** (Table 4-1).

DSM-IV general diagnostic criteria for personality disorders are outlined in Table 4-2. Criteria for individual personality disorders are discussed below. Personality disorders frequently overlap in symptoms.

CLUSTER A (ODD AND ECCENTRIC)

PARANOID PERSONALITY DISORDER

People with paranoid personality disorder are distrustful and suspicious and anticipate harm and betrayal.

Epidemiology

Paranoid personality disorder has a lifetime prevalence of 0.5% to 2.5% of the general population. Relatives of patients with chronic schizophrenia and patients with persecutory delusional disorders show an increased prevalence of paranoid personality disorder.

Etiology

Environmental precursors are unclear. Family studies suggest a link to delusional disorder (paranoid type). There appears to be a small increase in prevalence among relatives of individuals with schizophrenia.

Clinical Manifestations

History and Mental Status Examination

People with paranoid personality disorder are distrustful, suspicious, and see the world as malevolent. They anticipate harm, betrayal, and deception. Not surprisingly, they are not forthcoming about themselves. They require emotional distance.

Differential Diagnosis

The key distinction is to separate paranoia associated with psychotic disorders from paranoid personality disorder, especially because paranoia associated with psychotic disorders is generally responsive to antipsychotic medications.

SCHIZOID PERSONALITY DISORDER

Individuals with schizoid personality disorder are emotionally detached and prefer to be left alone.

Epidemiology

Estimates of lifetime prevalence range as high as 7.5% of the general population, but because people with schizoid personality disorder are avoidant of others, they are not commonly seen in clinical practice.

Etiology

There is some evidence to suggest increased prevalence of schizoid personality disorder in relatives of persons with schizophrenia or schizotypal personality disorder. Unloving or neglectful parenting is hypothesized to play a role.

TABLE 4-1 Personality Disorders 1: Classification of Personality Disorders		
Cluster A (Odd/ Eccentric)	Cluster B (Dramatic/ Emotional)	Cluster C (Anxious/ Fearful)
Paranoid	Antisocial	Avoidant
Schizoid	Borderline	Dependent
Schizotypal	Histrionic	Obsessive–
	Narcissistic	compulsive

Clinical Manifestations

History and Mental Status Examination

These people are loners. They are aloof and detached and have profound difficulty experiencing or expressing emotion. Although they prefer to be left alone and generally do not seek relationships, they may maintain an important bond with a family member.

Differential Diagnosis

Schizoid personality disorder can be distinguished from avoidant personality disorder (see below) and social phobia by the fact that schizoid individuals do not desire relationships. Avoidant and socially phobic persons desire and may seek relationships, but their

TABLE 4-2 General Diagnostic Criteria for Personality Disorders
Patients with personality disorder evidence an enduring pattern of inner experience and behavior, established by adolescence or early adulthood, that:
1. Deviates markedly from cultural expectations
2. Is inflexible and personally and socially pervasive
3. Causes distress or social or work impairment
4. Is a stable pattern of experience and behavior of long duration ("stably unstable")
5. Cannot be explained by another mental illness
6. Is not caused by substance use or medical condition
NOTE: Individuals with personality disorders usually maintain intact reality testing. However, they may have transient psychotic symptoms when stressed by real (or imagined) loss or frustration. Personality disorders are different from personality traits that are typically adaptive, culturally acceptable, and do not cause significant distress or impairment. *Source:* American Psychiatric Association, *Diagnostic and statistical manual of mental disorders,* 4th ed. Washington, DC: .American Psychiatric Association, 2000.

anxiety handicaps their capacity to achieve relatedness. Schizophrenia, autistic disorder, and Asperger's disorder (a less severe variant of autism) are also differential diagnostic conditions.

SCHIZOTYPAL PERSONALITY DISORDER

Individuals with schizotypal personality disorder have odd thoughts, affects, perceptions, and beliefs.

Epidemiology

Lifetime prevalence is 3% of the general population.

Etiology

Studies demonstrate interfamilial aggregation of this disorder, especially among first-degree relatives of individuals with schizophrenia.

Clinical Manifestations

History and Mental Status Examination

Schizotypal personality disorder is best thought of as similar to schizophrenia but less severe and without sustained psychotic symptoms. People with this disorder have few relationships and demonstrate oddities of thought, affect, perception, and belief. Many are highly distrustful and often paranoid, which results in a very constricted social world. The lifetime suicide rate among this population is 10%.

Differential Diagnosis

Schizophrenia, delusional disorder, and mood disorder with psychosis are the major differential diagnoses.

CLUSTER B (DRAMATIC AND EMOTIONAL)

ANTISOCIAL PERSONALITY DISORDER

Individuals with antisocial personality disorder (ASP) repetitively disregard the rules and laws of society and rarely experience remorse for their actions.

Epidemiology

Antisocial personality disorder is present in 3% of men and 1% of women. About half have been arrested; about half of those in prison have ASP.

Etiology

ASP is more common among first-degree relatives of those diagnosed with ASP. In families of an individual with ASP, men show higher rates of ASP and substance abuse, whereas women have higher rates of somatization disorder. A harsh, violent, and criminal environment also predisposes people to this disorder.

Clinical Manifestations

History and Mental Status Examination

Individuals with ASP display either a flagrant or well-concealed disregard for the rules and laws of society. They are exploitative, lie frequently, endanger others, are impulsive and aggressive, and rarely experience remorse for the harm they cause others. Alcoholism is a frequently associated finding in this population. Many individuals with ASP are indicted or jailed for their actions. Their lifetime suicide rate is 5%.

Differential Diagnosis

Bipolar disorder and substance abuse disorder can prompt antisocial behaviors during the acute illness, which remit when the disorder is controlled. The antisocial behavior of individuals with ASP, conversely, is not state dependent.

BORDERLINE PERSONALITY DISORDER

Individuals with borderline personality disorder suffer from instability in relationships, self-image, affect, and impulse control.

Epidemiology

Lifetime prevalence is 1% to 2% of the general population.

Etiology

Borderline personality disorder is about five times as common among first-degree relatives of borderline patients. In addition, this disorder shows increased rates in families of alcoholics and families of individuals with ASP, as well as in families with mood disorders. Females with borderline personality disorder frequently have suffered from sexual or physical abuse or both.

Clinical Manifestations

History and Mental Status Examination

Individuals with borderline personality disorder suffer from a legion of symptoms. Their relationships are infused with anger, fear of abandonment, and shifting idealization and devaluation. Their self-image is inchoate, fragmented, and unstable with consequent unpredictable changes in relationships, goals, and values. They are affectively unstable and reactive, with anger, depression, and panic prominent. Their impulsiveness can result in many unsafe behaviors, including drug use, promiscuity, gambling, and other risk-taking behavior. Their self-destructive urges result in frequent suicidal and parasuicidal behavior (such as superficial cutting or burning or nonfatal overdoses in which the intent is not lethal). They also demonstrate brief paranoia and dissociative symptoms. Suicide attempts can be frequent before the age of 30, and suicide rates approach 10% over a lifetime. The principal intrapsychic defenses such individuals use are primitive with gross denial, distortion, projection, and splitting prominent. Patients may exhibit a broad range of comorbid illnesses, including substance abuse, mood disorders, and eating disorders.

Differential Diagnosis

Mood disorders and behavioral changes due to active substance abuse are the principal differential diagnostic considerations. The diagnostic clues are unstable relationships, unstable self-image, unstable affect, and unstable or impulsive behaviors.

HISTRIONIC PERSONALITY DISORDER

Individuals with histrionic personality disorder have excessive superficial emotionality and a powerful need for attention.

Epidemiology

Lifetime prevalence is 2% to 3% of the general population. In clinical settings, the diagnosis is most frequently applied to women but may equally affect men in the general population.

Etiology

There appears to be a familial link to somatization disorder and to ASP.

Clinical Manifestations

History and Mental Status Examination

Individuals with histrionic personality disorder are characterized by their excessive and superficial emotionality and their profound need to be the center of attention at all times. Theatrical behavior dominates with lively and dramatic clothing, exaggerated emotional responses to seemingly insignificant events, and inappropriate flirtatious and seductive behavior across a wide variety of circumstances. Despite their apparent plethora of emotion, these individuals often have difficulty with intimacy, frequently believing their relationships are more intimate than they actually are.

Differential Diagnosis

Somatization disorder is the principal differential diagnostic consideration.

NARCISSISTIC PERSONALITY DISORDER

Individuals with narcissistic personality disorder appear arrogant and entitled but suffer from extremely low self-esteem.

Epidemiology

Lifetime prevalence is estimated at 1% in the general population and 2% to 16% in clinical populations. Up to 50% to 75% of those with this diagnosis are men.

Etiology

The etiology of this disorder is unknown.

Clinical Manifestations

History and Mental Status Examination

People with narcissistic personality disorder demonstrate an apparently paradoxical combination of self-centeredness and worthlessness. Their sense of self-importance is generally extravagant, and they demand attention and admiration. Concern or empathy for others is typically absent. They often appear arrogant, exploitative, and entitled. However, despite their inflated sense of self, below their brittle facade lies low self-esteem and intense envy of those whom they regard as more desirable, worthy, or able.

Differential Diagnosis

The grandiosity of narcissism can be differentiated from the grandiosity of bipolar disorder by the presence of characteristic mood symptoms in bipolar disorder.

CLUSTER C (ANXIOUS AND FEARFUL)

AVOIDANT PERSONALITY DISORDER

Individuals with avoidant personality disorder desire relationships but avoid them because of the anxiety produced by their sense of inadequacy.

Epidemiology

Lifetime prevalence is 0.5% to 1% of the general population and appears to be equally prevalent in men and women.

Etiology

There are no conclusive data. The pattern of avoidance may start in infancy.

Clinical Manifestations

History and Mental Status Examination

People with avoidant personality disorder experience intense feelings of inadequacy. They are painfully sensitive to criticism, so much so that they are compelled to avoid spending time with people. Their fears of rejection and humiliation are so powerful that to engage in a relationship they seek strong guarantees of acceptance. The essence of this disorder is inadequacy, hypersensitivity to criticism, and consequent social inhibition.

Differential Diagnosis

The major diagnostic distinction is between avoidant personality disorder and social phobia, generalized type.

DEPENDENT PERSONALITY DISORDER

Individuals with dependent personality disorder are extremely needy, relying on others for emotional support and decision-making.

Epidemiology

Lifetime prevalence is 15% to 20%, 2% to 3% clinically.

Etiology

The etiology is unknown.

Clinical Manifestations

History and Mental Status Examination

These people yearn to be cared for. Because of their extreme dependence on others for emotional support and decision-making, they live in great and continual fear of separation from someone they depend on, hence their submissive and clinging behaviors.

Differential Diagnosis

People with dependent personality disorder are similar to individuals with borderline personality disorder in their desire to avoid abandonment but do not exhibit the impulsive behavior, unstable affect, and poor self-image of the borderline patient.

OBSESSIVE–COMPULSIVE PERSONALITY DISORDER

These individuals are perfectionists who require a great deal of order and control.

Epidemiology

The estimated prevalence is 1% in the general population. Men are diagnosed with obsessive–compulsive personality disorder twice as frequently as women.

Etiology

The etiology is unknown, but there may be an association with mood and anxiety disorders.

Clinical Manifestations

History and Mental Status Examination

Individuals with obsessive–compulsive personality disorder are perfectionists. They require order and control in every dimension of their lives. Their attention to minutiae frequently impairs their ability to finish what they start or to maintain sight of their goals. They are cold and rigid in relationships and make frequent moral judgments; devotion to work often replaces intimacy. They are serious and plodding; even recreation becomes a sober task.

Differential Diagnosis

Obsessive–compulsive personality disorder can be differentiated from obsessive–compulsive disorder (OCD) based on symptom severity.

MANAGEMENT

Because personality may have temperamental components and is developed over a lifetime of interacting with the environment, personality disorders are generally resistant to treatment. In general, **psychotherapy** is recommended for most personality disorders. **Psychodynamically based therapies** are commonly used, although they must be modified to each individual and each disorder. **Cognitive, behavioral,** and **family therapies** are also used to treat these disorders. Empirical studies validating the efficacy of various therapies are generally lacking. **Dialectical behavioral therapy** (DBT) was developed specifically for the treatment of borderline personality disorder and has been validated in empirical studies. Group therapy incorporating various psychotherapeutic modalities is also used.

Pharmacotherapy is widely used in personality disorders, although no specific medication has been shown to treat any specific disorder. Instead, medications are targeted at the various associated symptoms of personality disorders. For example, mood stabilizers may be used for mood instability and impulsiveness. Benzodiazepines are commonly used for anxiety, although the potential for abuse and dependence is too often overlooked. Beta-blockers are also used frequently. For depression, obsessive–compulsive symptoms, and eating disturbances, selective serotonin-reuptake inhibitors (SSRIs) and other antidepressants have been successfully used. Psychotic or paranoid symptoms are commonly treated with low-dose antipsychotics.

🔑 4-1 KEY POINTS

1. Personality disorders are categorized into three symptom clusters.
2. Personality disorders consist of an enduring pattern of experience and behavior.
3. The disorders can produce transient psychotic symptoms during stress.
4. Treatment is with psychotherapy and medications targeted at symptom relief.
5. Personality disorders are resistant to treatment.
6. Personality disorders may have genetic associations with Axis I disorders.

References

Kool S, Schoevers R, de Maat S, et al. Efficacy of pharmacotherapy in depressed patients with and without personality disorders: a systematic review and meta-analysis. *J Affect Disord*. 2005 Nov; 88(3): 269–278.

Livesley WJ. Behavioral and molecular genetic contributions to a dimensional classification of personality disorder. *J Personal Disord*. 2005 Apr;19(2):131–155. Review.

Livesley WJ. Principles and strategies for treating personality disorder. *Can J Psychiatry*. 2005 Jul;50(8):442–450.

Paris J. Recent advances in the treatment of borderline personality disorder. *Can J Psychiatry*. 2005 Jul;50(8):435–441.

Substance-Related Disorders

Substance abuse is as common as it is costly to society. It is etiologic for many medical illnesses and is frequently comorbid with psychiatric illness. The *Diagnostic and Statistical Manual of Mental Disorders*, 4th edition (DSM-IV) defines substance abuse and dependence independent of the substance. Hence, alcohol abuse and dependence is defined by the same criteria as heroin abuse and dependence. This chapter defines abuse and dependence and provides clinical descriptions of each substance-related disorder. The DSM-IV recognizes the different signs and symptoms associated with various drug addictions. Here the common substance-related disorders are reviewed in sequence.

SUBSTANCE ABUSE

The DSM-IV defines substance abuse as a maladaptive pattern of substance use leading to clinically significant impairment or distress as manifested by one or more of the following:

- Failure to fulfill major role obligations at home, school, or work;
- Recurrent substance use in situations in which it is physically hazardous;
- Recurrent substance-related legal problems;
- Recurrent substance use despite persistent or recurrent social or interpersonal problems caused or exacerbated by the effects of the substance.

SUBSTANCE DEPENDENCE

Substance dependence is defined as a maladaptive pattern of substance use leading to clinically significant impairment or distress, as manifested by three or more of the following occurring at any time in a 12-month period:

1. Tolerance;
2. Withdrawal;
3. Repeated, unintended, excessive use;
4. Persistent failed efforts to cut down;
5. Excessive time spent trying to obtain the substance;
6. Reduction in important social, occupational, or recreational activities;
7. Continued use despite awareness that substance is the cause of psychological or physical difficulties.

Although each substance dependence disorder has unique features, these are considered the common features that define substance dependence. Major substance use disorders are discussed with particular attention to their unique features.

ALCOHOL-RELATED DISORDERS

ALCOHOL INTOXICATION

Alcohol intoxication is defined by the presence of slurred speech, incoordination, unsteady gait, nystagmus, impairment in attention or memory, stupor or coma, and clinically significant maladaptive behavioral or psychological changes (inappropriate sexual or aggressive behavior, mood lability, impaired judgment, impaired social or occupational functioning) that develops during or shortly after alcohol ingestion.

The diagnosis of alcohol intoxication must be differentiated from other medical or neurologic states that may mimic intoxication, for example, diabetic hypoglycemia; toxicity with various agents, including but not limited to ethylene glycol, lithium, and phenytoin; and intoxication with benzodiazepines or barbiturates. The diagnosis of alcohol intoxication can be confirmed by serum toxicologic screening, including a blood alcohol level (BAL).

ALCOHOL DEPENDENCE

Alcohol abuse becomes alcohol dependence when effects on one's life become more global and **tolerance** and **withdrawal** symptoms develop. The alcoholically dependent patient drinks larger amounts over longer periods of time than intended, spends a great deal of time attempting to obtain alcohol, and reduces participation in or eliminates important social, occupational, or recreational activities because of alcohol. In alcohol dependence, there also is a persistent desire or unsuccessful efforts to cut down or control alcohol intake.

Epidemiology

The percentage of Americans who abuse alcohol is thought to be high. Two thirds of Americans drink occasionally; 12% are heavy drinkers, drinking almost every day and becoming intoxicated several times a month. The Epidemiological Catchment Area study found a lifetime prevalence of alcohol dependence of 14%. The male–female prevalence ratio for alcohol dependence is 4:1.

Etiology

The etiology of alcohol dependence is unknown. Adoption studies and monozygotic twin studies demonstrate a partial genetic basis, particularly for men with alcoholism. Male alcoholics are more likely than female alcoholics to have a family history of alcoholism. Compared with control subjects, the relatives of alcoholics are more likely to have higher rates of depression and antisocial personality disorder (ASP). Adoption studies also reveal that alcoholism is multidetermined: genetics and environment (family rearing) both play a role.

Clinical Manifestations

History

The alcohol-dependent patient may deny or minimize the extent of drinking, making the early diagnosis of alcoholism difficult. The patient may present with accidents or falls, blackouts, motor vehicle accidents, or after an arrest for driving under the influence. Because denial is so prominent in the disorder, collateral information from family members is essential to the diagnosis. Early physical findings that suggest alcoholism include acne rosacea, palmar erythema, and painless hepatomegaly (from fatty infiltration).

Physical Examination

Signs of more advanced alcoholism include cirrhosis, jaundice, ascites, testicular atrophy, gynecomastia, and Dupuytren contracture. Cirrhosis can lead to complications including variceal bleeding, hepatocellular carcinoma, and hepatic encephalopathy. Medical disorders with an increased incidence in alcohol-dependent patients include pneumonia, tuberculosis, cardiomyopathy, hypertension, and gastrointestinal cancers (i.e., oral, esophageal, rectal, colon, pancreas, and liver).

Mental Status Examination

There are also numerous neuropsychiatric complications of alcoholism. **Wernicke–Korsakoff's syndrome** may develop in the alcohol-dependent patient because of **thiamine deficiency**. The Wernicke's stage of the syndrome consists of the triad of **nystagmus, ataxia**, and **mental confusion**; however, few patients with Wernicke's syndrome display the complete triad and the diagnosis of Wernicke's syndrome may be missed in up to 90% of clinical presentations. These symptoms remit with the slow intravenous infusion of thiamine at 400 to 500 mg per day for 4 to 5 days. Magnesium repletion is also essential. Without thiamine at sufficiently high dosages and given intravenously, Wernicke's encephalopathy may progress to Korsakoff's psychosis (**anterograde amnesia** and **confabulation**), which is irreversible in two thirds of patients. Other neuropsychiatric complications of alcoholism include alcoholic hallucinosis, alcohol-induced dementia, peripheral neuropathy, mental status changes due to subdural hematoma or other intracranial bleeding, substance-induced depression, and suicide. In the later stages of alcoholism, significant social and occupational impairment is likely: job loss and family estrangement are typical.

Laboratory Tests

Various laboratory tests are helpful in making the diagnosis. BALs quantitatively confirm alcohol in the serum. They can also provide a rough measure of tolerance. In general, the higher the BAL without significant signs of intoxication, the more tolerant the patient has become of the intoxicating effects of alcohol.

Alcohol-dependent patients also develop elevated high-density lipoprotein cholesterol and decreased low-density lipoprotein cholesterol, elevated mean corpuscular volume, elevated serum glutamic-oxaloacetic transaminase, and elevated serum glutamic-pyruvic transaminase. Of alcohol-dependent patients, 30%, compared with 1% of control subjects, have evidence of old rib fractures on chest radiographs.

Differential Diagnosis

The diagnosis of alcohol dependence is usually clear after careful history, physical and mental status examination, and consultation with family or friends.

Management

Management is specific to the clinical syndrome. Alcohol intoxication is treated with supportive measures, including decreasing external stimuli and withdrawing the source of alcohol. Intensive care may be required in cases of excessive alcohol intake complicated by respiratory compromise. All suspected or known alcohol-dependent patients should receive oral vitamin supplementation with folate 1 mg per day and thiamine 100 mg per day. If oral intake is not possible, thiamine should be administered intravenously as a slow infusion before any glucose is given (because glucose depletes thiamine stores).

Alcohol withdrawal syndromes include the following.

Minor Withdrawal

"The shakes" begin 12 to 18 hours after cessation of drinking and peak at 24 to 48 hours. Untreated, uncomplicated alcohol withdrawal lasts 5 to 7 days. It is characterized by tremors, nausea, vomiting, tachycardia, and hypertension. Minor withdrawal is treated with benzodiazepines, such as chlordiazepoxide (Librium) or oxazepam (Serax) titrated to the degree of withdrawal signs. The benzodiazepine is then tapered over a period of days. The goals of treatment are prevention of more serious complications and patient comfort.

Major Withdrawal

The risk of alcoholic seizures ("rum fits") begins 7 to 36 hours after cessation of drinking and peaks between 24 and 48 hours. One to six generalized seizures are common but rarely lead to status epilepticus. Alcoholic seizures precede delirium tremens in 30% of cases. Seizures are treated acutely with intravenous benzodiazepines. Prophylactic phenytoin (Dilantin) may be effective when administered during the high-risk period in patients with a history of withdrawal seizures.

Alcoholic hallucinosis has an onset within 48 hours of cessation of drinking and may last more than a week. It is characterized by vivid, unpleasant auditory hallucinations in the presence of a clear sensorium. Alcoholic hallucinosis may be treated with an antipsychotic (e.g., haloperidol or an atypical antipsychotic medication). On rare occasions, these hallucinations become chronic.

Alcohol withdrawal delirium (delirium tremens) is a life-threatening condition manifested by delirium (perceptual disturbances, confusion or disorientation, agitation), autonomic hyperarousal, and mild fever. It affects up to 5% of hospitalized patients with alcohol dependence and typically begins 2 to 3 days after abrupt reduction in or cessation of alcohol intake. It is treated with intravenous benzodiazepines and supportive care. Treatment may need to occur in an intensive care unit, particularly if there is significant autonomic instability (e.g., rapidly fluctuating blood pressure). The syndrome typically lasts 3 days but can persist for weeks.

Alcohol Rehabilitation

The two goals of rehabilitation are **sobriety** and treatment of **comorbid psychopathology**.

To sustain a lasting recovery, the patient must stop denying the illness and accept the diagnosis of alcohol dependence. Alcoholics Anonymous (AA), a worldwide self-help group for recovering alcohol-dependent patients, has been shown to be one of the most effective programs for achieving and maintaining sobriety. The program involves daily to weekly meetings that focus on 12 steps toward recovery. Members are expected to pursue the 12 steps with the assistance of a sponsor (preferably someone with several years of sobriety).

Alcohol appears to be a potent cause of depression. Intoxicated patients may appear severely depressed and display suicidal behavior or statements, which resolve when sobriety is achieved. Treatment of depression should be geared to patients who remain depressed after 2 to 4 weeks of sobriety. Anxiety is also common in withdrawing or newly sober patients and should be assessed after at least 1 month of sobriety. Inpatient and residential rehabilitation programs use a team approach aimed at focusing the patient on recovery. Group therapy allows patients to see their own problems mirrored in and confronted by others. Family therapy allows the patient to examine the role of the family in alcoholism.

Disulfiram (Antabuse) can be helpful in maintaining sobriety in some patients. It acts by inhibiting the second enzyme in the pathway of alcohol metabolism, aldehyde dehydrogenase, so that acetaldehyde accumulates in the bloodstream, causing flushing, nausea, vomiting, palpitations, and hypotension. In theory, disulfiram should inhibit drinking by making it physiologically unpleasant; however, because the effects can be fatal in rare cases, patients must be committed to abstinence and fully understand the danger of drinking while taking disulfiram. The usual dose of disulfiram is 250 mg daily.

Naltrexone (Revia) is an opiate antagonist medication. Naltrexone reduces both the amount of alcohol intake and the frequency of alcohol intake. Naltrexone is usually dosed at 50 mg per day, but higher doses may potentially be more effective. Unlike disulfiram, patients can continue taking naltrexone if they relapse to alcohol intake. Naltrexone, as an opioid antagonist, may work in part by reducing the reinforcing "high" of alcohol ingestion.

Acamprosate (Campral) is a glutamate receptor modulator (and may also affect gamma-amino butyric acid, GABA) medication used for the maintenance of alcohol abstinence and in reducing the rate and severity of relapse. Like naltrexone, acamprosate does not produce a disulfiram-like effect and can be continued in persons who relapse to alcohol consumption.

It is important to note that disulfiram, naltrexone, and acamprosate are used for **maintenance** therapy and do not prevent the potentially life-threatening symptoms of alcohol withdrawal.

Many studies have demonstrated benefits from rehabilitation programs, but nearly half of all treated alcohol-dependent patients will relapse, most commonly in the first 6 months.

🔑 5-1 KEY POINTS

1. In alcohol dependence, denial and minimization are common.
2. Benzodiazepines are used in acute detoxification to prevent life-threatening complications of withdrawal.
3. Peak incidence of alcoholic seizures is within 24 to 48 hours.
4. Rehabilitation is aimed at abstinence and treating comorbid disorders.
5. Rehabilitation involves AA and group and family therapies.
6. Of treated alcoholics, 50% will relapse.
7. Wernicke–Korsakoff's syndrome is due to thiamine deficiency.
8. Wernicke's triad consists of nystagmus, ataxia, and mental confusion.
9. Korsakoff's symptoms are anterograde amnesia and confabulation.

SEDATIVE, HYPNOTIC, AND ANXIOLYTIC SUBSTANCE USE DISORDERS

Sedative, hypnotic, and anxiolytic drugs are widely used. They are all **cross-tolerant** with each other and with alcohol. Included in this class are barbiturates and benzodiazepines. Of these, the benzodiazepines are the most widely prescribed and available.

EPIDEMIOLOGY

Approximately 15% of the general population is prescribed a benzodiazepine in a given year. Some patients abuse these drugs.

CLINICAL MANIFESTATIONS

History

Sedative-hypnotic drug abuse and dependence are associated with syndromes of intoxication, withdrawal, and withdrawal delirium that resemble those of alcohol.

Physical and Mental Status Examinations

Intoxication only can be distinguished from alcohol intoxication by the presence (or absence) of alcohol on the breath, or in the serum or urine. Barbiturates, when taken orally, are much more likely than benzodiazepines to cause clinically significant respiratory compromise.

Laboratory Tests

Intoxication can be confirmed through quantitative or qualitative serum or urine toxicologic analyses. Serum toxicologic screens can identify the presence of benzodiazepines and barbiturates and their major metabolites.

Withdrawal symptoms are listed in Table 5-1. Withdrawal delirium (confusion, disorientation, and visual and somatic hallucinations) has an onset of 3 to 4 days after abstinence. Dependence requires the presence of three or more of the seven symptoms listed in Table 5-1.

MANAGEMENT

Treatment of sedative-hypnotic withdrawal may be on an outpatient or inpatient basis. Generally, inpatient detoxification is required when there is comorbid medical or psychiatric illness, prior treatment failures,

■ TABLE 5-1 Signs and Symptoms of Sedative-Hypnotic Withdrawal	
Minor Withdrawal	**More Severe Withdrawal**
Restlessness	Coarse tremors
Apprehension	Weakness
Anxiety	Vomiting
	Sweating
	Hyperreflexia
	Nausea
	Orthostatic hypotension
	Seizures

or lack of support by family or friends. On an inpatient unit, benzodiazepines or barbiturates may be administered and tapered in a controlled manner. Withdrawal from short-acting substances is generally more severe, whereas withdrawal from longer-acting substances is more prolonged.

Withdrawal from barbiturates is more dangerous than from benzodiazepines: it can (much more easily) lead to hyperpyrexia and death. Withdrawal is managed by scheduled dosing and tapering of a benzodiazepine or barbiturate (diazepam or phenobarbital).

In patients who have been abusing alcohol and benzodiazepines or barbiturates, it may be necessary to perform a **pentobarbital challenge test**. This test allows for the quantification of tolerance to perform a controlled taper, thereby reducing the problems of withdrawal.

Treatment of sedative-hypnotic dependence resembles that for alcohol dependence. After detoxification, the patient can enter a residential rehabilitation program or a day or evening treatment program. Referral to AA is appropriate because the addiction issues and recovery process are similar. Families may be referred to Al-Anon, an AA focused family education and support group.

⚷ 5-2 KEY POINTS

1. Sedatives and hypnotic drugs are cross-tolerant with alcohol.
2. The agents have intoxicating effects and result in withdrawal states similar to alcohol.
3. Tolerance can be measured by a pentobarbital challenge test.
4. Treatment resembles that for alcoholism.

OPIOID USE DISORDERS

Opiates include morphine, heroin, codeine, meperidine, and hydromorphone. Heroin is available only illegally in the United States. Opiates are commonly used for pain control.

EPIDEMIOLOGY

Opiate use and abuse are relatively uncommon in the United States. Past year prevalence for heroin dependence in 2003 was 0.1% and past year prevalence for prescription pain reliever dependence was 0.6%. Many of those who use opiates recreationally become addicted.

CLINICAL MANIFESTATIONS

History

Most heroin and morphine users take opiates intravenously, which produces flushing and an intensely pleasurable, diffuse bodily sensation that resembles orgasm. This initial "rush" is followed by a sense of well-being. Psychomotor retardation, drowsiness, inactivity, and impaired concentration ensue.

Physical and Mental Status Examinations

Signs of intoxication occur immediately after the addict "shoots up" and include pupillary constriction, respiratory depression, slurred speech, hypotension, bradycardia, and hypothermia. Nausea, vomiting, and constipation are common after opiate use.

Laboratory Tests

Opiate use can be confirmed by urine or serum toxicologic measurements.

Opiate abuse is defined by the criteria for substance abuse noted above. In opiate dependence, tolerance to the effects of opiates occurs. Addicts "shoot up" three or more times per day.

Withdrawal symptoms usually begin 10 hours after the last dose. Withdrawal from opiates can be highly uncomfortable but is rarely medically complicated or life-threatening. Withdrawal symptoms are listed in Table 5-2.

Opiate addicts often have comorbid substance use disorders, antisocial or borderline personality disorders, and mood disorders. Opiate addicts are more prone to

TABLE 5-2 Symptoms of Opiate Withdrawal

Mild Withdrawal	More Severe Withdrawal
Dysphoric mood, anxiety, and restlessness	Nausea
	Vomiting
Lacrimation or rhinorrhea	Muscle aches
Pupillary dilatation	Seizures (in meperidine withdrawal)
Piloerection	
Sweating	Abdominal cramps
Tachycardia	Hypertension
Fever	Hot and cold flashes
Diarrhea	Severe anxiety
Insomnia	
Yawning	

commit crimes because of the high cost of opiates. Opiate addiction also is associated with high mortality rates from inadvertent overdoses, accidents, and suicide. Opiate addicts are also at higher risk of medical problems because of poor nutrition and use of dirty needles. Common medical disorders include serum hepatitis, human immunodeficiency virus (HIV) infection, endocarditis, pneumonia, and cellulitis.

Differential Diagnosis

The diagnosis of opiate addiction is usually obvious after a careful history and mental status and physical examinations.

MANAGEMENT

Patients addicted to opiates should be gradually withdrawn using methadone. **Methadone** is a weak agonist of the *mu* opiate receptor and has a longer half-life (15 hours) than heroin or morphine. Thus, it causes relatively few intoxicant or withdrawal effects. Generally, the initial dose of methadone (typically 5 to 20 mg) is based on the profile of withdrawal symptoms. Withdrawal from short-acting opiates lasts 7 to 10 days; withdrawal from longer-acting meperidine lasts 2 to 3 weeks.

Buprenorphine (Buprenex) is a *mu* opioid receptor partial agonist and a kappa opioid receptor antagonist. Injectable buprenorphine is employed as an off-label use for opiate detoxification. Buprenorphine

tablets as Subutex (buprenorphine alone) or as Suboxone (buprenorphine plus naltrexone) are FDA approved for outpatient treatment of opioid dependence by certain qualified physicians. Approval of the tablet form of buprenorphine permitted the expansion of the treatment of opioid dependence beyond that of methadone clinics. Inclusion of naltrexone with buprenorphine in Suboxone allows the administration of opiate replacement therapy with decreased euphoric and respiratory depressant effects.

Clonidine, a centrally acting alpha 2 receptor agonist that decreases central noradrenergic output, can also be used for acute withdrawal syndromes. It is remarkably effective at treating the autonomic symptoms of withdrawal but does little to curb the drug craving. Risks of sedation and hypotension limit the usefulness of clonidine in outpatient settings. Clonidine does not appear to be as effective as opiate replacement in helping maintain abstinence. Additional medications can be used to relieve uncomfortable symptoms of withdrawal, such as dicyclomine for abdominal cramping, promethazine for nausea, and quinine for muscle aches.

Rehabilitation generally involves referral to an intensive day treatment program and to Narcotics Anonymous, a 12-step program similar to AA. Methadone maintenance, daily administration of 60 to 100 mg of methadone in government-licensed methadone clinics, is used widely for patients with demonstrated physiologic dependence. Long-term administration of methadone can alleviate drug hunger and minimize drug-seeking behavior.

🔑 5-3 KEY POINTS

1. Recreational use of opiates often leads to addiction.
2. Opiate addicts are at increased risk of HIV, pneumonia, endocarditis, hepatitis, and cellulitis.
3. High mortality occurs from accidental overdose, suicide, and accidents.
4. Opiate withdrawal begins 10 hours after last dose.
5. Withdrawal is uncomfortable but not usually medically complicated.

CENTRAL NERVOUS SYSTEM STIMULANT USE DISORDERS

Cocaine and amphetamines are readily available in the United States. The patterns of use and abuse of and dependence on cocaine and amphetamines are similar because both are **central nervous system (CNS) stimulants** with similar psychoactive and sympathomimetic effects.

In the United States, cocaine is available in two forms: as cocaine hydrochloride powder, which is typically snorted, and as cocaine alkaloid crystal ("crack"), which is typically smoked. Cocaine has an extremely rapid onset of action (when snorted or smoked) and a short half-life, requiring frequent dosing to remain "high."

In the United States, an amphetamine (dextroamphetamine) and methylphenidate are available in pill form by prescription for the treatment of obesity, narcolepsy, and attention-deficit/hyperactivity disorder. Various forms of amphetamine are used illicitly including a very pure form of methamphetamine, called crystal methamphetamine, which can be snorted or smoked. Amphetamines have a longer half-life than cocaine and hence are taken less frequently.

Rates of depression are generally higher in substance-abusing and substance-dependent individuals. Antidepressant medications influencing catecholamine function, such as desipramine and bupropion, are generally superior to the SSRIs in the treatment of cocaine-related depression.

CLINICAL MANIFESTATIONS

Cocaine or amphetamine intoxication is characterized by:

1. Maladaptive behavioral changes (e.g., euphoria or hypervigilance);
2. Tachycardia or bradycardia;
3. Pupillary dilatation;
4. Hyper- or hypotension;
5. Perspiration or chills;
6. Nausea or vomiting;
7. Weight loss;
8. Psychomotor agitation or retardation;
9. Muscular weakness, respiratory depression, chest pain, cardiac dysrhythmias;
10. Confusion, seizures, dyskinesia, or coma.

Cocaine intoxication can cause tactile hallucinations ("coke bugs"). Both cocaine and amphetamine intoxication can lead to agitation, impaired judgment, and **transient psychosis** (e.g., paranoia, visual hallucinations). Cocaine and amphetamine dependence is defined by the criteria outlined above for substance dependence.

Withdrawal of cocaine or amphetamines leads to fatigue, depression, nightmares, headache, profuse sweating, muscle cramps, and hunger. Withdrawal symptoms peak in 2 to 4 days.

MANAGEMENT

Withdrawal from amphetamines or other CNS stimulants is self-limited and usually does not require inpatient detoxification. Psychosis from amphetamine intoxication or withdrawal is generally self-limited, requiring only observation in a safe environment. Antipsychotic medications can be used to treat agitation.

Ultimately, the goal is rehabilitation. Narcotics Anonymous, treatment of comorbid psychopathology, administration of drugs to reduce craving, and family therapy are the essential features of cocaine rehabilitation.

🔑 5-4 KEY POINTS

1. Cocaine and amphetamines are CNS stimulants.
2. CNS stimulants can cause transient psychosis (e.g., "coke bugs" or paranoia).
3. Withdrawal symptoms (fatigue, depression, nightmares, etc.) peak in 2 to 4 days.
4. Withdrawal from CNS stimulants is self-limited.

CANNABIS AND MISCELLANEOUS SUBSTANCE USE DISORDERS

CANNABIS

Cannabis is widely used throughout the world in the forms of marijuana and hashish. The drug is usually smoked and causes a state of euphoria. Complications of cannabis include impaired judgment, poor concentration, and poor memory. Serious complications include delirium and psychosis.

CLUB DRUGS

Club Drugs are a group of drugs classified by the National Institute on Drug Abuse (NIDA) according to their popularity in dance clubs and other party venues. These drugs are of a wide variety of chemical classes, but are linked by their frequent use in social groups and the fact that they are commonly taken together. Because of their popularity and tendency for users to show up in emergency rooms, we review some of the more widely used club drugs below.

Ecstasy (MDMA)—Ecstasy is a widely popular drug with mixed stimulant and hallucinogenic properties. Many users report a stimulant and euphoric effect, and MDMA appears specifically to enhance the user's desire for intimacy with others. As such, its use has been associated with an increased frequency of unsafe sexual activity. Acute use of MDMA has been associated with deaths from various causes. Long-term MDMA use appears to lead to a permanent loss of fine-diameter serotonin axons throughout the brain.

Methamphetamine—Also known as crystal or crank, methamphetamine is a psychostimulant that is neurotoxic to dopamine and serotonin axons. Methamphetamine is often produced locally in small laboratories and can therefore vary greatly in purity.

Gamma-Hydroxybutyrate (GHB)—GHB is a compound used in lower doses by bodybuilders and others seeking to gain muscle mass (GHB promotes the release of growth hormone). In higher doses, GHB is used to produce a high, and is common among the club and party scene. GHB is easily overdosed, and can lead to death from respiratory arrest.

Ketamine—Also known as Special K, ketamine is a dissociative anesthetic mostly used in veterinary medicine. It is used for its hallucinatory, dissociative effect.

Rohypnol—Rohypnol is a benzodiazepine approved for clinical use in some countries outside the United States. Rohypnol produces classic benzodiazepine effects of sedation. However, it has strong amnestic properties, and may be a frequent culprit in drugging others for the purpose of theft or sexual assault.

Lysergic acid diethylamide (LSD)—LSD is famous for its hallucinogenic properties. Acute use can produce a highly euphoric ("good trip") or a highly dysphoric ("bad trip") hallucinatory experience. Long-term LSD use can lead to psychosis or hallucinogen persisting perception disorder.

References

Cami J, Farre M. Drug addiction. *N Engl J Med.* 2003 Sep 4;349(10):975–986.

Fiellin DA, Kleber H, Trumble-Hejduk JG, et al. Consensus statement on office-based treatment of opioid dependence using buprenorphine. *J Subst Abuse Treat.* 2004 Sep;27(2):153–159.

Room R, Babor T, Rehm J. Alcohol and public health. *Lancet.* 2005 Feb 5–11;365(9458): 519–530.

Rounsaville BJ. Treatment of cocaine dependence and depression. *Biol Psychiatry.* 2004 Nov 15;56(10):803–809.

Thomson AD, Cook CC, Touquet R, et al, and Royal College of Physicians, London. The Royal College of Physicians report on alcohol: guidelines for managing Wernicke's encephalopathy in the accident and Emergency Department. *Alcohol Alcoholism.* 2002 Nov–Dec;37(6):513–521.

Eating Disorders

Eating disorders are characterized by disturbances in eating behavior and an overconcern with body image or size. Although eating disorders are classified into two discrete diagnostic categories in the *Diagnostic and Statistical Manual of Mental Disorders*, 4th edition (DSM-IV), many symptoms overlap. The principal diagnostic distinction is based on ideal body weight. When abnormal eating behavior causes body weight to fall below a defined percentage of expected body weight, a diagnosis of anorexia nervosa is made. If ideal body weight is maintained in the presence of abnormal eating behaviors, a diagnosis of bulimia nervosa is made. Eating disorders likely lie along a continuum of disturbances in eating behavior and often are associated with mood disorders and other psychiatric illnesses (Table 6-1).

ANOREXIA NERVOSA

Anorexia nervosa is a severe eating disorder characterized by **low body weight**. Anorexia nervosa is diagnosed when a person's body weight falls below 85% of the ideal weight for that individual. The weight loss must be due to behavior directed at maintaining low weight or achieving a particular body image.

EPIDEMIOLOGY

The point prevalence of anorexia nervosa is between 0.5% and 1% in women, and more than 90% of patients with anorexia nervosa are women. The prevalence in men is not clear. Average age of onset is 17, with onset rare before puberty or after age 40. Anorexia nervosa is more common in industrial societies and higher socioeconomic classes.

ETIOLOGY

Eating disorders and their subtypes likely share many common bases of origin. Psychological theories of anorexia nervosa remain speculative. Patients with anorexia nervosa generally have a high fear of losing control, difficulty with self-esteem, and commonly display "all or none" thinking. Although it is not specific to eating disorders, past physical or sexual abuse may be a risk factor. Contemporary theories focus on the need to control one's body.

Social theories propose that societal opinions, which equate low body weight with attractiveness, drive women to develop eating disorders. Although this fact may be responsible for some cases (e.g., anorexia nervosa is more common among dancers and models), historically anorexia nervosa has been present during periods when societal mores for beauty were different.

Biologic, familial, and genetic data support a biologic and heritable basis for anorexia. Family studies reveal an increased incidence of mood disorders and anorexia nervosa in first-degree relatives of patients with anorexia nervosa. Twin studies show higher concordance for monozygotic versus dizygotic twins. Neuroendocrine evidence supporting a biologic contribution to anorexia includes alterations in corticotropin-releasing factor, reduced central nervous system norepinephrine metabolism, and that amenorrhea (caused by decreased luteinizing hormone and follicle-stimulating hormone release) sometimes precedes the onset of anorexia nervosa.

CLINICAL MANIFESTATIONS

History and Mental Status Examination

DSM-IV criteria for the diagnosis of anorexia nervosa include refusal to keep body weight at greater than 85%

■ TABLE 6-1 Classification of Eating Disorders	
Anorexia Nervosa	Bulimia Nervosa
Restricting type	Nonpurging type
Binge eating/purging type	Purging type

of ideal, an intense fear of weight gain, preoccupation with body size and shape, a disproportionate influence of body weight on personal worth, and the denial of the medical risks of low weight. Patients with anorexia nervosa generally do not have a loss of appetite; they refuse to eat out of fear of gaining weight. Amenorrhea is also a diagnostic criterion in postmenarchal females (delay of menarche may occur in premenarchal girls). In some cases, amenorrhea precedes the development of anorexia nervosa; however, in most cases, it appears to be a consequence of starvation.

Individuals with anorexia nervosa commonly exercise intensely to lose weight and alter body shape. Some restrict food intake as a primary method of weight control; others use binging and purging (use of laxatives, enemas, diuretics, or induced vomiting) to control weight.

The behavioral repertoire used to control body weight is used to classify anorexia nervosa further into two subtypes: restricting type and binging/purging type. In the restricting type, the major methods of weight control are food restriction and exercise. In the binging/purging type, food restriction and exercise may be present, but binge eating and subsequent purging behaviors also are present.

The natural course of anorexia is not well understood, but many cases become chronic. The long-term mortality of anorexia nervosa secondary to suicide or medical complications is greater than 10%.

Differential Diagnosis

Conditions that can resemble anorexia should be ruled out. These include major depression with loss of appetite and weight, some psychotic disorders where nutrition may not be adequate, body dysmorphic disorder, and a variety of general medical (especially neuroendocrine) conditions. Anorexia nervosa is differentiated from bulimia nervosa by the presence of low weight in individuals with the former.

Management

The management of anorexia nervosa is directed at the presenting symptoms. When medical complications are present, these must be carefully treated and followed. If ipecac use to induce vomiting is suspected, ipecac toxicity must be ruled out.

During starvation, psychotherapy is of little value because of the cognitive impairment produced by starvation. When patients are less medically ill, a therapeutic program including supervised meals; weight and electrolyte monitoring; psychoeducation about the illness, starvation, and nutrition; individual psychotherapy, and family therapy can begin. Psychopharmacology management often includes antidepressants, especially the selective serotonin reuptake inhibitors (SSRIs) to treat comorbid depression. Psychopharmacologic treatments are used principally to treat any comorbid psychiatric illness and have little or no effect on the anorexia per se.

🔑 6-1 KEY POINTS

1. Anorexia nervosa is a severe eating disorder characterized by low body weight.
2. The disorder is diagnosed more than 90% of the time in women.
3. Anorexia nervosa can cause serious medical complications and has a greater than 10% long-term mortality rate.

BULIMIA NERVOSA

Bulimia nervosa is an eating disorder characterized by **binge eating** with the **maintenance of body weight**.

EPIDEMIOLOGY

The estimated point prevalence of bulimia nervosa is 1% to 3% of women. The male–female ratio is 1:10. This illness occurs disproportionately among whites in the United States.

ETIOLOGY

Many of the factors in the genesis of anorexia nervosa are also implicated in bulimia nervosa. Familial and genetic studies support similar familial linkages in both disorders. Psychological theories for bulimia nervosa stress an addiction or obsessive–compulsive behavioral model. Biologic, neurologic, and endocrine findings are less prominent in theories of causation of bulimia nervosa. Abnormal serotonin metabolism is thought to play more of a role in bulimia nervosa than in anorexia nervosa.

CLINICAL MANIFESTATIONS

History and Mental Status Examination

Bulimia nervosa is diagnosed in individuals who engage in binge eating and behaviors designed to avoid weight gain but who maintain their body weight. In addition, these are people whose self-evaluation is overly influenced by their body weight and shape.

Food binges in bulimia nervosa may be precipitated by stress or altered mood states. Once a binge begins, the individual typically feels out of control and continues to eat large quantities of food, often to the point of physical discomfort. **Purging** may follow and most often consists of vomiting, usually induced mechanically by stimulating the gag reflex or using ipecac. Other purging methods used to avoid weight gain include laxative and diuretic abuse and enemas. Individuals with bulimia often exercise and restrict their food intake. As in anorexia nervosa, patients with bulimia nervosa are overly concerned with body image and are preoccupied with becoming fat. Bulimia nervosa is classified into two subtypes: nonpurging type or purging type (Table 6-1) according to whether purging behavior is present.

Differential Diagnosis

Bulimia nervosa should be distinguished from the binge eating and purging subtype of anorexia nervosa. If body weight is less than 85% of ideal, a diagnosis of anorexia nervosa is made. Binge eating can occur in major depression and in borderline personality disorder, but is not tied to a compulsion to reduce weight.

MANAGEMENT

The treatment for bulimia nervosa is similar to that for anorexia nervosa. Although medical complications of starvation are not present, other medical complications can require careful medical management and, at times, hospitalization. Psychotherapy focuses at first on achieving control of eating behavior. Cognitive therapy may be useful in treating overconcern with body image. Self-esteem and interpersonal relationships become the focus of therapy as the behavioral

problems abate. Antidepressants, especially SSRIs, are more effective in the treatment of bulimia nervosa than in anorexia nervosa (including those patients who do not have comorbid depression).

🔑 6-2 KEY POINTS

1. Bulimia nervosa is a severe eating disorder characterized by binge eating and purging.
2. The disorder is also characterized by maintenance of normal body weight.
3. Bulimia nervosa is more common in women than in men.
4. Bulimia nervosa can have serious medical complications.

■ TABLE 6-2 Medical Complications of Eating Disorders

Behavior	Medical Complication
Binge eating	Gastric dilatation or rupture
	Obesity
Vomiting	Esophageal rupture
	Parotiditis with hyperamylasemia
	Hypokalemic, hypochloremic, metabolic alkalosis (with cardiac arrhythmias)
	Ipecac toxicity (cardiac and skeletal myopathies)
Laxative use	Constipation (due to laxative dependence)
	Metabolic acidosis
	Dehydration
Diuretic use	Electrolyte abnormalities (with cardiac arrhythmias)
	Dehydration
Starvation	Leukopenia, anemia
	Increased ventricular/brain ratio
	Hypotension, bradycardia
	Hypothermia
	Hypercholesterolemia
	Edema
	Dry skin, lanugo hair

MEDICAL COMPLICATIONS

Eating disorders, when persistent, can have serious medical consequences. The lifetime mortality from anorexia nervosa is approximately 10%; it is unknown for bulimia nervosa. Table 6-2 lists the common medical complications of eating disorders. The most serious of these, gastric or esophageal rupture, cardiomyopathy from ipecac toxicity, and cardiac arrhythmias secondary to electrolyte imbalance, can be fatal. Other complications parallel those of chronic medical illness, take a severe toll on the patient's overall functioning, and cause tremendous suffering and burden for their families. In addition to these medical complications, secondary psychiatric and neurologic sequelae include cognitive decline, metabolic encephalopathy, and severe mood disturbance, all with profound consequences for patients and their families.

References

Fairburn CG. Evidenced-based treatment of anorexia nervosa. *Int J Eating Disorder.* 2005;37 (Suppl):S26–S30.

Lilly RZ. Bulimia nervosa. *Br Med J.* 2003;327: 380–381.

Disorders of Childhood and Adolescence

Many disorders seen in adults can occur in children. However, there is a group of disorders usually first diagnosed in children. Table 7-1 lists these disorders according to the *Diagnostic and Statistical Manual of Mental Disorders*, 4th edition (DSM-IV). This chapter reviews only the more common disorders.

Child psychiatric assessment requires attention to details of a child's stage of development, family structure and dynamics, and normative age-appropriate behavior. Consulting with parents and obtaining information from schools, teachers, and other involved parties (e.g., Department of Social Services/Youth Services) are essential to proper assessment.

Children, especially young children, usually express emotion in a more **concrete** (less abstract) way than adults. Consequently, child interviews require more concrete queries (Do you feel like crying? *instead of* Are you sad?). Playing games, taking turns telling stories, and imaginative play are often used to gain insight into the child's emotional and interpersonal life. During play, observations are also made regarding activity level, motor skills, and verbal expression. Children are much more likely than adults to have **comorbid** mental disorders, making diagnosis and treatment more complicated.

The complexities of diagnosis in child psychiatry often require the use of psychological testing. Tests of general intelligence include the Stanford-Binet Intelligence Scale (one of the first intelligence tests developed and often used in young children) and the Wechsler Intelligence Scale for Children–Revised (WISC-R). The WISC-R is the most widely used intelligence test for assessing school-age children. It yields a verbal score, a performance score, and a full-scale score (both verbal and performance) or **intelligence quotient (IQ)**.

There are many other tests and objective rating scales designed to measure behavior (e.g., impulsiveness, physical activity), perceptual-motor skills (by drawing people, placing pegs in appropriately shaped holes), and personality style (by describing what is happening in an ambiguous scene).

Because seizure activity or subtle electroencephalographic abnormalities are common in certain child psychiatric disorders, an **electroencephalogram (EEG)** may be warranted. The evaluation of mental retardation usually involves a search for possible causes.

MENTAL RETARDATION

Patients with mental retardation have subnormal intelligence (as measured by IQ) combined with deficits in adaptive functioning. IQ is defined as the mental age (as assessed using a WISC-R) divided by the chronologic age and multiplied by 100. If mental age equals chronologic age, then the ratio equals 1 and the IQ is "100." An IQ of less than 70 is required for the diagnosis of mental retardation. Severity ranges from mild to profound and is based on IQ (Table 7-2).

EPIDEMIOLOGY

Mental retardation affects 1% to 2% of the population and has a male–female ratio of 2:1. Milder forms of mental retardation occur more frequently in families with low socioeconomic status (SES); more severe forms of mental retardation are independent of SES. Most patients with mental retardation have mild or moderate forms (Table 7-2).

ETIOLOGY

Mental retardation can be thought of as a final common pathway of a number of childhood or perinatal

■ **TABLE 7-1** Disorders Usually First Diagnosed in Infancy, Childhood, or Adolescence

Mental Retardation

Learning Disorders

   Reading Disorder

   Mathematics Disorder

   Disorder of Written Expression

Motor Skills Disorder

   Developmental Coordination Disorder

Communication Disorders

   Expressive Language Disorder

   Mixed Receptive-Expressive Language Disorder

   Phonological Disorder

   Stuttering

Pervasive Developmental Disorders

   Autistic Disorder

   Rett's Disorder

   Childhood Disintegrative Disorder

   Asperger's Disorder

Attention-Deficit and Disruptive Behavior Disorders

   Attention-Deficit/Hyperactivity Disorder

   Conduct Disorder

   Oppositional Defiant Disorder

Feeding and Eating Disorders of Infancy or Early Childhood

   Pica

   Rumination Disorder

   Feeding Disorder of Infancy or Early Childhood

Tic Disorders

   Tourette's Disorder

   Chronic Motor or Vocal Tic Disorder

   Transient Tic Disorder

Elimination Disorders

   Encopresis

   Enuresis

Other Disorders of Infancy, Childhood, or Adolescence

   Separation Anxiety Disorder

   Selective Mutism

   Reactive Attachment Disorder of Infancy or Early Childhood

   Stereotypic Movement Disorder

■ **TABLE 7-2** Mental Retardation

Degree of MR	IQ	Percentage of Total MR Population
Mild	50–70	85%
Moderate	35–50	10%
Severe	20–35	3%–4%
Profound	<20	1%–2%

disorders. The most common cause of mental retardation is **Down's syndrome** (trisomy 21). **Fragile X syndrome** is the most common cause of *heritable* mental retardation. Inborn errors of metabolism; perinatal or early childhood head injuries; maternal diabetes, substance abuse, toxemia, or rubella can all cause mental retardation. Overall, there are more than 500 genetic abnormalities associated with mental retardation. In 30% to 40% of patients with mental retardation, no clear etiology can be determined.

CLINICAL MANIFESTATIONS

History, Physical and Mental Status Examinations, and Laboratory Tests

Most mentally retarded children have physical malformations that identify them at birth as being at high risk for mental retardation (such as the characteristic facies of the child with Down's syndrome). Infants can show signs of significantly subaverage intellectual functioning. Young children with mental retardation may be identified by parents or pediatricians after failure to meet developmental milestones in a number of functional areas (e.g., delayed speech, social skills, or self-care skills capacity) or on scoring an IQ less than 70 on the Stanford-Binet (usually only for very young children) or WISC–R (standard for school-age children).

The onset of symptoms must be before age 18. The patient must have both an IQ less than or equal to 70 and concurrent deficits or impairments in several areas of adaptive functioning (e.g., communication, self-care, interpersonal skills). Laboratory findings may suggest metabolic or chromosomal etiology.

Differential Diagnosis

Attention-deficit/hyperactivity disorder (ADHD), learning disorders, depression, schizophrenia, and seizure disorder can all resemble mental retardation. These disorders can also be comorbid conditions. Children suspected of having mental retardation should have a thorough medical and neurologic evaluation, including IQ testing, an EEG, and brain imaging (computerized tomography, CT, or magnetic resonance imaging, MRI).

MANAGEMENT

Management depends on the degree of retardation, the course, and the particular abilities of the child and the parents. Most children with mental retardation progress through normal milestones (standing, walking, talking, learning to recognize letters and numbers) in a pattern similar to normal children but at a slower rate. Growth and development occur in children with mental retardation. They can have developmental spurts, like normal children, that could not have been predicted at an earlier age.

In mild mental retardation, the child is typically considered educable. The child can usually learn to read, write, and perform simple arithmetic. With family support and special education, most of these children will be able to live with their parents. The long-term goal of treatment is to teach the child to function in the community and to hold some type of job.

In moderate mental retardation, the child is typically considered trainable. With training, the child can learn to talk, to recognize his or her name and a few simple words, and to perform activities of daily living (bathing, dressing, handling small change) without assistance. The long-term goal of treatment is typically to enable the child to live and function in a supervised group home.

Children with severe or profound mental retardation almost invariably require care in institutional settings, usually beginning very early in life. These forms of mental retardation are often associated with specific syndromes (e.g., Tay-Sachs's disease) in which there is progressive physical deterioration leading to premature death.

🔑 7-1 KEY POINTS

1. Mental retardation is defined by IQ less than or equal to 70 and impaired functioning in specific areas.
2. The condition is more common in males (2:1).
3. Mental retardation is most commonly caused by Down's syndrome (trisomy 21).
4. Mental retardation is managed in developmentally appropriate settings.

LEARNING DISORDERS

Learning disorders are characterized by performance in a specific area of learning (e.g., reading, writing, arithmetic) substantially below the expectation of a child's chronologic age, measured intelligence, and age-appropriate education. The DSM-IV identifies three learning disorders: **reading disorder, mathematics disorder**, and **disorder of written expression**.

ETIOLOGY

Specific learning disorders often occur in families. They are presumed to result from **focal cerebral injury** or from a **neurodevelopmental defect**.

EPIDEMIOLOGY

Learning disorders are relatively common. Reading disorder affects 4% of school-age children and mathematics disorder is estimated at 1%. The incidence of disorder of written expression is not yet known. Learning disorders are two to four times more common in boys than girls.

CLINICAL MANIFESTATIONS

History, Mental Status Examination, and Laboratory Tests

Specific learning disorders are typically diagnosed after a child has exhibited difficulties in a specific academic area. Because reading and arithmetic are usually not taught before the first grade, the diagnosis is seldom made in preschoolers. Some children may not be diagnosed until fourth or fifth grade, particularly if they have a high IQ and can mask their deficits. The diagnosis of learning disorder is confirmed through specific intelligence and achievement testing. Children with learning disorders do not obtain achievement test scores consistent with their overall IQs.

Differential Diagnosis

It is important to establish that a low achievement score is not due to some other factor such as lack of opportunity to learn, poor teaching, or cultural factors (e.g., English as a second language). Physical factors (such as hearing or vision impairment) must also be ruled out.

Finally, it is important to consider and test for more global disorders such as pervasive developmental disorder, mental retardation, and communication disorders. It is not uncommon to find that several of these disorders coexist. A specific learning disorder diagnosis is made when the full clinical picture is not adequately explained by other comorbid conditions.

MANAGEMENT

Children with these disorders often need remedial education, especially if their diagnosis was made late. They also need to be taught learning strategies to overcome their particular deficits. Acceptable skills in the disordered area can often be achieved with steady supportive educational assistance, although patients may be affected by these disorders throughout adulthood.

🔑 7-2 KEY POINTS

1. There are three types of learning disorders: mathematics, reading, and written expression.
2. The disorders tend to be familial and are probably due to cerebral injury or maldevelopment.
3. Reading disorder is the most common and all three disorders occur more often in boys (2:1 to 4:1).
4. The diagnosis is confirmed through achievement tests.
5. Physical or social factors must be ruled out.
6. Management involves remedial education and learning strategies.

PERVASIVE DEVELOPMENTAL DISORDERS

The DSM-IV groups **autistic disorder, Rett's disorder, childhood disintegrative disorder**, and **Asperger's disorder** under the heading of pervasive developmental disorders. These conditions are also referred to as autism spectrum disorders because of overlapping aspects of their clinical manifestations.

AUTISTIC DISORDER

Autistic disorder is a common pervasive developmental disorder of childhood onset. It is characterized by the triad of impaired social interactions, impaired ability to communicate, and restricted repertoire of activities and interests.

ETIOLOGY

Autistic disorder is familial. Genetic studies demonstrate incomplete penetrance (36% concordance rate in monozygotic twins), although a specific genetic defect has not been discovered. A small percentage of those with autistic disorder have a fragile X chromosome, and a high rate of autism exists with **tuberous sclerosis.**

EPIDEMIOLOGY

Autistic disorder is rare. It occurs in 2 to 5 children per 10,000 live births. The male–female ratio is 3:1 to 4:1.

CLINICAL MANIFESTATIONS

History, Mental Status Examination, and Laboratory Tests

Abnormal development is usually first noted soon after birth. Commonly, the first sign is **impairment in social interactions** (failure to develop a social smile, facial expressions, or eye-to-eye gaze). Older children often fail to develop nonverbal forms of communication (e.g., body postures and gestures) and may seem to have no desire or to lack the skills to form friendships. There is also a lack of seeking to share enjoyment (i.e., not showing, sharing, or pointing out objects they find interesting). By definition, findings must be present before age 3.

Autistic disorder is also characterized by a **marked impairment in communication**. There may be delay in or total lack of language development. Those children who do develop language show impairment in the ability to initiate and sustain conversations and use repetitive or idiosyncratic language. Language may also be abnormal in pitch, intonation, rate, rhythm, or stress.

Finally, there are usually **restrictive, repetitive, or stereotyped patterns of behavior, interests, or activities**. There may be an encompassing preoccupation with one or more stereotyped and restricted patterns of interest (e.g., amassing baseball trivia), an inflexible adherence to specific nonfunctional routines or rituals (e.g., eating the same meal in the same place at the same time each day), stereotyped or repetitive motor mannerisms (e.g., whole-body rocking), and a persistent preoccupation with the parts of objects (e.g., buttons).

Approximately 25% of children with autistic disorder have comorbid seizures; approximately 75%

have mental retardation (the moderate type is most common). EEGs and intelligence testing are typically part of the initial evaluation. Rarely, specific special skills are present, e.g., calendar calculation.

Differential Diagnosis

The diagnosis is usually clear after careful history, mental status examination, and developmental monitoring. However, childhood psychosis, mental retardation (alone), language disorders, and congenital deafness or blindness must all be ruled out.

MANAGEMENT

Autistic disorder is a chronic lifelong disorder with relatively severe morbidity. Very few individuals with autism will ever live independently. Once the diagnosis is made, parents should be informed that their child has a neurodevelopmental disorder (not a behavioral disorder that they might feel responsible for creating). The parents will have to learn **behavioral management techniques** designed to reduce the rigid and stereotyped behaviors of the disorder and improve social functioning. Many children with autism require special education or specialized day programs for behavior management.

Children with autism with a comorbid seizure disorder are treated with anticonvulsants. Low doses of **neuroleptics** (e.g., haloperidol) and some mood stabilizers and antidepressants have been shown to help decrease aggressive or self-harming behaviors.

RETT'S DISORDER

Rett's disorder is a pervasive developmental disorder that is a major cause of mental retardation in girls.

ETIOLOGY

The precise etiology of Rett's disorder is not known for all cases but the condition has been most commonly linked to mutations in the gene encoding methyl-CpG-binding protein 2 (MeCP2). Neuropathologically, Rett's disorder is associated with microcephaly with increased neuronal density but a decrease in neuronal dendrites and synaptic density in some brain regions.

EPIDEMIOLOGY

Rett's disorder occurs almost exclusively in females. The condition occurs in about 1 in every 15,000 births.

CLINICAL MANIFESTATIONS

History, Mental Status Examination, and Laboratory Tests

Children with Rett's syndrome appear normal for several months after birth and then develop specific problems. The precise DSM-IV diagnostic criteria require normal head circumference at birth, normal prenatal and perinatal development, and normal psychomotor development through the first 5 months after birth. Following this period of normalcy, there is a decrease in the rate of head growth between months 5 and 48; loss of acquired hand skills between 5 and 30 months (with the onset of stereotyped hand wringing/hand washing-like movements); loss of social engagement early in the illness (that may improve later); poorly coordinated gait or trunk movements; and severe impairments in language development with severe psychomotor retardation. Comorbid severe mental retardation and seizure disorder are common (but mental retardation and seizure are not part of the DSM-IV diagnostic criteria).

There are no laboratory tests for the diagnosis of Rett's disorder although genotyping may reveal associated mutations. Other conditions must be ruled out.

Differential Diagnosis

The differential diagnostic conditions primarily include other pervasive developmental disorders such as autistic disorder, childhood disintegrative disorder, and Asperger's disorder.

MANAGEMENT

Management is largely via behavioral techniques and treatment of complications. Anti-seizure medications, antipsychotic medications, and other psychotropic medications may play a role in managing behavioral difficulties.

CHILDHOOD DISINTEGRATIVE DISORDER

Childhood disintegrative disorder is characterized by a period of normal development followed by loss of function in multiple domains. It is the rarest of the pervasive developmental disorders.

ETIOLOGY

The etiology of childhood disintegrative disorder is unknown. The condition can be associated with general medical conditions affecting the brain.

EPIDEMIOLOGY

The condition is quite rare and much less common than autism. There may be a preponderance of males.

CLINICAL MANIFESTATIONS

History, Mental Status Examination, and Laboratory Tests

The DSM-IV diagnostic criteria for childhood disintegrative disorder require apparently normal childhood development for the first 2 years of life followed by a loss of previously acquired skills before age 10. Previously acquired skills can be lost in the domains of language, social skills and adaptive behavior, bowel or bladder control, play and motor skills. Additionally, there may be impaired functioning in social interaction or communication, or the development of restricted or repetitive behaviors, interests, and activities. The course is usually chronic once loss of skills has stabilized. This condition usually co-occurs with mental retardation and increased rates of seizure disorder. Laboratory tests are aimed primarily at the exclusion of potentially treatable conditions affecting brain function.

Differential Diagnosis

The differential diagnostic conditions primarily include other pervasive developmental disorders such as autistic disorder, Rett's disorder, and Asperger's disorder. Treatable medical conditions affecting brain function should be ruled out.

MANAGEMENT

Management consists primarily of treatment for behavioral difficulties and associated conditions (e.g., seizure disorder).

ASPERGER'S DISORDER

Asperger's disorder may be the most common pervasive developmental disorder (but prevalence figures are controversial) and is characterized by impaired social interactions and restrictive, repetitive, and stereotyped behaviors and interest.

ETIOLOGY

The etiology of Asperger's disorder remains unknown. There is some familial contribution and numerous genetic, metabolic, and infectious factors have been considered.

EPIDEMIOLOGY

The incidence of Asperger's disorder varies with diagnostic method but is estimated as 4 per 1,000 children and is approximately four times more common in males. Half of all children with Asperger's disorder may not be diagnosed with the condition.

CLINICAL MANIFESTATIONS

History, Mental Status Examination, and Laboratory Tests

The DSM-IV diagnostic features of Asperger's disorder include impairments in social interaction (consisting of severe deficits in multiple nonverbal communication behaviors such as eye-to-eye gaze, facial expression, and body language) and peer relationships, decreased sharing of personal experiences with others, and decreased reciprocal social/emotional interaction. Additionally, there are repetitive and stereotyped behaviors and interests, such as preoccupation with stereotyped restricted patterns of interest; a rigid adherence to routines or rituals having little functional use; motor mannerisms and stereotypies; a focus or preoccupation on parts of objects. In Asperger's disorder, there are no delays in language or cognitive, self-help, environmental curiosity, or adaptive behavior domains. The course is usually chronic.

Differential Diagnosis

The differential diagnostic conditions primarily include other pervasive developmental disorders such as autistic disorder, Rett's disorder, and childhood disintegrative disorder.

MANAGEMENT

Treatment for Asperger's disorder is nonspecific and consists of educational, behavioral, and psychotherapeutic approaches targeted at maximizing social interactions. Pharmacologic treatment may be indicated for specific behaviors or comorbid conditions.

ATTENTION-DEFICIT/HYPERACTIVITY DISORDER

ADHD is characterized by a persistent and dysfunctional pattern of overactivity, impulsiveness, inattention, and distractibility.

ETIOLOGY

The disorder runs in families and cosegregates with mood disorders, substance use disorders, learning disorders, and antisocial personality disorder. Families with a child diagnosed with ADHD are more likely than those without ADHD offspring to have family members with the above-mentioned disorders.

The etiology of the disorder is unknown, but perinatal injury, malnutrition, and substance exposure have all been implicated. Many children with ADHD have abnormalities of sleep architecture (decreased rapid eye movement latency, increased delta latency), EEG, and soft neurologic signs. Brain imaging studies indicate that overall brain volume is smaller in children diagnosed with ADHD when compared with controls.

EPIDEMIOLOGY

The prevalence of ADHD in school-age children is estimated to be 3% to 5%. The boy–girl ratio ranges from 4:1 in the general population to 9:1 in clinical settings. Boys are much more likely than girls to be brought to medical attention.

CLINICAL MANIFESTATIONS

History, Mental Status Examination, and Laboratory Tests

To meet criteria for ADHD, a child must evidence the onset of inattentive or hyperactive symptoms before age 7; symptoms must also be present in two or more settings (e.g., school, home). Symptoms in only one setting suggest an environmental or psychodynamic cause.

Preschool-age children are usually brought for evaluation when they are unmanageable at home. Typically, they stay up late, wake up early, and spend most of their waking hours in various hyperactive and impulsive activities. Children with a great deal of hyperactivity may literally run about the house, cause damage, and wreak havoc.

When these children enter school, their difficulties with attention become more obvious. They appear not to follow directions, forget important school supplies, fail to complete homework or in-class assignments, and attempt to blurt out answers to teachers' questions before being called on. As a result of their inattention and hyperactivity, these children often become known as "troublemakers." They fall behind their peers academically and socially.

Evaluation of the child involves gathering a careful history from parents and teachers (the latter usually through report cards and written reports). The child's behavior with and without the parent is carefully observed during psychiatric assessment. Informal testing is carried out by having the child attempt to complete a simple puzzle, write the letters of the alphabet, distinguish right from left, and recognize letters traced on the palms (graphesthesia). Physical examination, particularly focusing on neurologic function, is imperative. No specific laboratory or cognitive tests are helpful in making the diagnosis.

Differential Diagnosis

It is important to distinguish symptoms of ADHD from age-appropriate behaviors in active children (running about, being noisy, etc.). Children can also appear inattentive if they have a low or a high IQ and the environment is overstimulating or understimulating, respectively. In either instance, IQ testing and careful evaluation of the school program will clarify the diagnosis.

Children with oppositional defiant disorder may resist work or school tasks because of an unwillingness to comply with others' demands but not out of difficulty in attention.

Children with other mental disorders (e.g., mood disorder, anxiety disorder) can exhibit inattention but typically not before age 7. The child's history of school adjustment is not usually characterized by teacher or parent reports of inattentive, disruptive behavior.

Symptoms that resemble ADHD can occur in children before age 7, but the etiology is typically a side effect of a medication (e.g., bronchodilators) or a psychotic or pervasive developmental disorder; these children are not considered to have ADHD. Of course, ADHD may be comorbid with any of the above disorders. A dual diagnosis is made only when it is needed to explain the full clinical picture.

MANAGEMENT

The management of ADHD involves a combination of somatic and behavioral treatments. Most children with ADHD respond favorably to **psychostimulants**. Methylphenidate is the first-line agent, followed by D-amphetamine. Clinicians try to use the smallest effective dose and to restrict use to periods of greatest need (i.e., the school day) because psychostimulants have undesirable long-term physical effects (weight loss and inhibited body growth). Some children can be treated effectively with agents that raise norepinephrine in the brain, such as bupropion (Wellbutrin) or atomoxetine (Strattera), a norepinephrine reuptake inhibitor.

Behavioral management techniques include positive reinforcement, firm limit setting, and techniques for reducing stimulation (e.g., one playmate at a time; short, focused tasks).

CONDUCT DISORDER AND OPPOSITIONAL DEFIANT DISORDER

Conduct disorder is defined as a repetitive and persistent pattern of behavior in which the basic rights of others or important age-appropriate societal norms or rules are violated. Disordered behaviors include aggression toward people or animals, destruction of property, deceitfulness, theft, or serious violations of rules (school truancy, running away). Conduct disorder is the childhood equivalent of adult antisocial personality disorder (ASP). It is the most common disorder seen in outpatient psychiatric clinics and is frequently seen comorbidly with ADHD or learning disorders. Adoption studies show a genetic predisposition, but psychosocial factors play a major role. Parental separation or divorce, parental substance abuse, severely poor or inconsistent parenting, and association with a delinquent peer group have been shown to have some relationship to the development of conduct disorder.

Treatment involves individual and family therapy. Some children may need to be removed from the home and placed in foster care. Parents who retain custody of a child with conduct disorder are taught limit setting, consistency, and other behavioral techniques. Medications are used only to treat a comorbid ADHD or mood disorder but not for the conduct disorder itself. The long-term outcome depends on the severity of the disorder and the degree and type of comorbidity. Of children with conduct disorder, 25% to 40% go on to have adult ASP.

Oppositional defiant disorder is diagnosed in a child with annoying, difficult, or disruptive behavior when the frequency of the behavior significantly exceeds that of other children his or her mental age (or that is less tolerated in the child's particular culture). It is a relatively new diagnosis that is meant to describe children with behavior problems that do not meet criteria for full-blown conduct disorder. Management emphasizes individual and family counseling.

🔑 7-4 KEY POINTS

1. ADHD is characterized by inattentiveness and hyperactivity occurring in multiple settings.
2. Symptoms must begin before age 7.
3. ADHD is more common in boys (4:1).
4. For a diagnosis of ADHD, other causes of inattentiveness or hyperactivity must be ruled out.
5. ADHD is managed with psychostimulants and behavioral techniques.

🔑 7-5 KEY POINTS

1. Conduct disorder is the childhood equivalent of ASP.
2. The disorder is defined by observable measurable behaviors.
3. Conduct disorder is the most common diagnosis in outpatient child psychiatric clinics.
4. The disorder is managed by limit-setting, consistency, and behavioral techniques.
5. Oppositional defiant disorder is a less severe form of conduct disorder.

TOURETTE'S DISORDER

Tourette's disorder is a rare disorder in which the child demonstrates multiple involuntary motor and vocal tics. A **tic** is a sudden, rapid, recurrent, nonrhythmic, stereotyped motor movement or vocalization.

EPIDEMIOLOGY

Tourette's disorder affects 0.4% of the population. There is a 3:1 male–female ratio.

ETIOLOGY

Tourette's disorder is highly familial and appears to frequently co-occur with obsessive–compulsive disorder. Despite evidence of genetic transmission in some families, no gene (or genes) has yet been discovered to explain the etiology of the disorder.

CLINICAL MANIFESTATIONS

History, Mental Status and Physical Examinations

The patient or family usually describes an onset in childhood or early adolescence before age 18. Vocal tics are usually loud grunts or barks but can involve shouting words; the words are sometimes obscenities (coprolalia). The patient describes being aware of shouting the words, being able to exert some control over them, but being overwhelmed by an uncontrollable urge to say them. Motor tics can involve facial grimacing, tongue protrusion, blinking, snorting, or larger movements of the extremities or whole body. Motor tics typically antedate vocal tics; barks or grunts typically antedate verbal shouts. The motor tics are not painful.

Differential Diagnosis

A careful neurologic evaluation should be performed to rule out other causes of tics. Wilson's disease and Huntington's disease are the principal differential diagnostic disorders. An EEG should be performed to rule out a seizure disorder. Careful evaluation for other comorbid psychiatric illnesses should be performed. Stimulants used to treat other psychiatric disorders may unmask tics.

MANAGEMENT

Treatment for more severe tics typically involves the use of low doses of high-potency neuroleptics such as haloperidol or pimozide, but various other agents are used. The child and his or her family should receive education and **supportive psychotherapy** aimed at minimizing the negative social consequences (e.g., embarrassment, shame, isolation) that occur with this disorder.

🔑 7-6 KEY POINTS

1. Tourette's disorder is a tic disorder.
2. The disorder is rare and more common in males (3:1).
3. When diagnosing Tourette's disorder, Wilson's and Huntington's diseases must be ruled out.
4. Treatment is with high-potency neuroleptics and patient/family support.

CHILDHOOD FEEDING AND EATING DISORDERS

PICA

Pica is a condition characterized by the developmentally inappropriate ingestion of nonnutritive substances for a period of at least 1 month, when the ingestion of nonnutritive substances is not part of a culturally sanctioned behavior. Little is known about the etiology and epidemiology of pica. In the mentally retarded, rates of pica increase with increasing severity of mental retardation. Medical complications such as lead poisoning, gastrointestinal complications, and infectious consequences may result. The disorder may be sustained or self-limited.

RUMINATION DISORDER

Rumination disorder is a feeding disorder characterized by repeated regurgitation of ingested food for at least 1 month after a period of normal eating. The regurgitative behavior cannot be due to gastrointestinal difficulties or another eating disorder such as bulimia nervosa. The condition appears rare and is most commonly diagnosed in infants, but may appear at a later age in mentally retarded individuals. Regurgitated food may be expelled or re-chewed and swallowed. If regurgitation is severe and insufficient calories are ingested, malnutrition can occur. Mortality rates may approach 25%. Spontaneous remission is common. The etiology is unknown.

FEEDING DISORDER OF INFANCY OR EARLY CHILDHOOD

Feeding disorder is characterized by continued failure to eat enough food, leading to weight loss or failure to gain weight and lasting at least 1 month. The condition cannot be due to a general medical condition. Associated conditions such as those resulting from malnutrition with impaired sleep, irritability, and developmental delays may occur. The etiology is unclear but impaired caregiver–child interactions may play a role.

⚷ 7-7 KEY POINTS

1. There are three types of feeding and eating disorders of infancy or early childhood: pica, rumination disorder, and feeding disorder.
2. Pica is characterized by the developmentally inappropriate eating of nonnutritive substances such as dirt.
3. Rumination disorder is characterized by repeated regurgitation of ingested food in the absence of gastrointestinal or other medical pathology that develops after 1 month of normal eating.
4. Feeding disorder of infancy or early childhood is characterized by at least 1 month of failure to eat enough to maintain or gain weight in the absence of other medical causes.

ELIMINATION DISORDERS

ENCOPRESIS

The diagnostic criteria for encopresis require repeated episodes (at least once per month for at least 3 months) of defecation in inappropriate places in individuals at least 4 years old or having an equivalent developmental level. The inappropriate defecation cannot be due to another medical condition or drug with the exception of constipation. About 1% of 5-year-olds display encopresis. When present, encopresis is classified according to whether or not there is constipation with overflow incontinence.

ENURESIS

The diagnostic criteria for enuresis require repeated episodes (two times per week for at least 3 consecutive months or the presence of significant distress) of urination into one's clothes or bed in children at least 5 years old or having an equivalent developmental level. The inappropriate urination cannot be due to a general medical condition or substance. Enuresis is classified according to the time of day of occurrence as nocturnal only, diurnal only, or nocturnal and diurnal. About 7% of 5-year-old boys have enuresis. The prevalence is about 3% in 5-year-old girls.

⚷ 7-8 KEY POINTS

1. There are two types of elimination disorders: encopresis and enuresis.
2. Encopresis is characterized by repeated episodes of inappropriate defecating, such as in one's clothing, on the floor, etc.
3. Encopresis is classified according to the presence or absence of constipation with overflow incontinence.
4. Enuresis is characterized by repeated episodes of inappropriate urination, for example, into one's clothes or bed.
5. Enuresis is classified according to the time of day of occurrences as nocturnal only, diurnal only, or both nocturnal and diurnal.

References

Bridge Denckla M. ADHD: topic update. *Brain Dev.* 2003 Sep;25(6):383–389.

Khouzam HR, El-Gabalawi F, Pirwani N, et al. Asperger's disorder: a review of its diagnosis and treatment. *Compr Psychiatry.* 2004 May–Jun;45(3):184–191.

McClellan JM, Werry JS. Evidence-based treatments in child and adolescent psychiatry: an inventory. *J Am Acad Child Adolesc Psychiatry.* 2003 Dec;42(12): 1388–1400.

Neul JL, Zoghbi HY. Rett's syndrome: a prototypical neurodevelopmental disorder. *Neuroscientist.* 2004 Apr;10(2):118–128.

Chapter 8

Cognitive Disorders

The cognitive disorders are delirium, dementia, and amnestic disorders. Table 8-1 lists the *Diagnostic and Statistical Manual of Mental Disorders*, 4th edition, classification of cognitive disorders.

DELIRIUM

Delirium is a reversible state of global cortical dysfunction characterized by alterations in **attention** and **cognition** and produced by a definable precipitant. Delirium is categorized by its etiology (Table 8-1) as due to general medical conditions, as substance-related, or as multifactorial in origin.

ETIOLOGY

Delirium is a syndrome with many causes. The neurotransmitter most commonly implicated in delirium is acetylcholine. Excess central nervous system (CNS) acetylcholine is thought to cause delirium. However, alterations in other neurotransmitters such as gamma-amino butyric acid (GABA) and dopamine are also implicated. Most frequently, delirium is the result of a general medical condition; substance intoxication and withdrawal also are common causes. Structural CNS lesions can also lead to delirium. Table 8-2 lists common general medical and substance-related causes of delirium. Delirium is often multifactorial and may be produced by a combination of minor illnesses and minor metabolic derangements (e.g., mild anemia, mild hyponatremia, mild hypoxia, and urinary tract infection, especially in an elderly person). Common medical causes of delirium include metabolic abnormalities such as hyponatremia, hypoxia, hypercapnia, hypoglycemia, and hypercalcemia. Infectious illnesses, especially urinary tract infections, pneumonia, and meningitis, are often implicated. The common substance-induced causes of delirium are alcohol or benzodiazepine withdrawal and benzodiazepine and anticholinergic drug toxicity, although a great number of commonly used medications, both prescribed and available over the counter, can produce delirium. Other conditions predisposing to delirium include old age, fractures, and pre-existing dementia. Brain damage of any kind, whether associated with overt dementia, prior trauma, or ischemic changes, is a risk factor for the development of delirium.

EPIDEMIOLOGY

The exact prevalence of delirium in the general population is unknown. Delirium occurs in 10% to 15% of general medical patients older than age 65 and is frequently seen postsurgically and in intensive care units. Delirium is equally common in men and women.

CLINICAL MANIFESTATIONS

History and Mental Status Examination

History is critical in the diagnosis of delirium, particularly in regard to the time course of development of the delirium and to the prior existence of dementia or other psychiatric illness. Key features of delirium are as follows:

1. Disturbance of consciousness, especially attention and level of arousal;
2. Alterations in cognition, especially memory, orientation, language, and perception;
3. Development over a period of hours to days; and
4. Presence of medical or substance-related precipitants.

TABLE 8-1 Cognitive Disorders		
Delirium	**Dementia**	**Amnestic**
General medical	Alzheimer's type	General medical
Substance-related	Vascular origin	Substance-related
Multifactorial	HIV-related	
	Head trauma-related	
	Parkinson's-related	
	Huntington's-related	
	Pick's-related	
	Creutzfeldt–Jakob-related	
	General medical origin	
	Substance-related	
	Multifactorial	

TABLE 8-2 Common Causes of Delirium	
General Medical	**Substance-Related**
Infectious	Intoxication
Urinary tract infections	Alcohol
Meningitis	Hallucinogens
Pneumonia	Opioids
Sepsis	Marijuana
Metabolic	Stimulants
Hyponatremia	Sedatives
Hepatic encephalopathy	Withdrawal
Hypoxia	Alcohol
Hypercarbia	Benzodiazepines
Hypoglycemia	Barbiturates
Fluid imbalance	Medication-induced
Uremia	Anesthetics
Hypercalcemia	Anticholinergics
Postsurgical	Meperidine
Hyper/hypothyroidism	Antibiotics
Ictal/postictal	Toxins
Head trauma	Carbon monoxide
Miscellaneous	Organophosphates
Fat emboli syndrome	
Thiamine deficiency	
Anemia	

In addition, sleep–wake cycle disturbances and psychomotor agitation may occur. Delirium is often difficult to distinguish from dementia, in part because dementia is a risk factor for delirium (and thus they frequently co-occur) and in part because there is a great deal of symptom overlap, as outlined in Table 8-3. Key differentiating factors are the time course of development of the mental status change (especially if the patient did not have a prior dementia) and the presence of a likely precipitant for the mental status change. Individuals with delirium may also display periods of complete lucidity interspersed with periods of confusion, whereas in dementia the deficits are generally more stable. In both conditions, there may be nocturnal worsening of symptoms with increased agitation and confusion ("sundowning").

The available evidence suggests that there are subtypes of delirium identifiable via clinical observation of psychomotor activity. These can be characterized as hypoactive, hyperactive, and mixed deliria. Further research is needed to validate these subtypes and develop subtype-specific treatment strategies. However, an assessment for possible delirium in a quiet, or hypoactive patient, may be critical in the overall medical treatment of such a patient.

The diagnosis of delirium is complicated by the fact that there are no definitive tests for delirium.

The workup for delirium includes a thorough history and mental status examination, a physical examination, and laboratory tests targeted at identifying general medical and substance-related causes. These should include urinalysis, complete chemistry panel, complete blood count, and oxygen saturation. Additional workup might entail chest radiographs, arterial blood gas (ABG) assessment, neuroimaging, or electroencephalogram (EEG). EEG may reveal nonspecific diffuse slowing. The presence of a delirium is associated with a 1-year mortality rate of 40% to 50%.

Differential Diagnosis

Delirium should be differentiated from dementia (although both can be present at the same time), psychotic or manic disorganization, and status complex partial epilepsy.

■ TABLE 8-3 Delirium versus Dementia

	Delirium	Dementia
Onset	Hours to days	Weeks to years
Course/duration	Fluctuates within a day; may last hours to weeks[a]	Stable within a day; may be permanent, reversible, or progressive over weeks to years
Attention	Impaired	May be impaired
Cognition	Impaired memory, orientation, language	Impaired memory, orientation, language, executive function
Perception	Hallucinations, delusions, misinterpretations	Hallucinations, delusions
Sleep/wake	Disturbed, may have complete day/night reversal	Disturbed, may have no pattern
Mood/emotion	Labile affect	Labile affect; mood disturbances
Sundowning	Frequent	Frequent
Identified precipitant	Likely precipitant is present	Identifiable precipitant not required

[a]DSM-IV does not specify a limit for the duration for delirium; clinical experience suggests resolution within days to weeks, in most cases.

MANAGEMENT

The treatment of delirium involves keeping the patient safe from harm while addressing the delirium. In the case of delirium due to a general medical illness, the underlying illness must be treated; in substance-related delirium, treatment involves removing the offending drug (either drugs of abuse or medications) or the appropriate replacement and tapering of a cross-reacting drug to minimize withdrawal. Delirium in elderly individuals is frequently multifactorial and requires correction of a multitude of medical conditions.

In addition to addressing the cause of a delirium as the mainstay of treatment, oral, intramuscular, or intravenous haloperidol is of great use in treating delirium-associated agitation. Atypical antipsychotic medications are also used. However, there are no treatments for delirium approved by the U.S. Food and Drug Administration (FDA). While alcohol or benzodiazepine withdrawal delirium is treated in part with benzodiazepines, benzodiazepines may worsen or precipitate delirium arising from other causes. Providing the patient with a brightly lighted room with orienting cues such as names, clocks, and calendars is also useful.

⚷ 8-1 KEY POINTS

1. Delirium is a disorder of attention and cognition.
2. Delirium is likely due to alterations in multiple neurotransmitters.
3. There are hypoactive, hyperactive, and mixed subtypes.
4. Delirium has an abrupt onset and a variable course.
5. Delirium has an identifiable precipitant.
6. The 1-year mortality rate is greater than 40%.

DEMENTIA

Dementia is characterized by the presence of **memory impairment** in the presence of other **cognitive defects**. Dementia is categorized according to its etiology (Table 8-1). It can arise as a result of a specific disease, for example, Alzheimer's disease or human immunodeficiency virus (HIV) infection; a general medical condition; or a substance-related condition; or it can have multiple etiologies. The definitive cause may not be determined until autopsy.

ETIOLOGY

Generally, the etiology of dementia is brain neuronal loss that may be due to neuronal degeneration or to cell death secondary to trauma, infarction, hypoxia, infection, or hydrocephalus. Table 8-1 lists the major discrete illnesses known to produce dementia. In addition, there are a large number of general medical, substance-related, and multifactorial causes of dementia.

EPIDEMIOLOGY

The prevalence of dementia of all types is about 2% to 4% after age 65, increasing with age to a prevalence of about 20% after age 85. Specific epidemiologic factors relating to disease-specific causes of dementia are listed in Table 8-4.

CLINICAL MANIFESTATIONS

History and Mental Status Examination

Dementia is diagnosed in the presence of multiple cognitive defects not better explained by another diagnosis. The presence of memory loss is required; in addition, one or more cognitive defects in the categories of aphasia, apraxia, agnosia, and disturbance in executive function must be present. Table 8-3 compares characteristics of dementia with those of delirium. Dementia often develops insidiously over the course of weeks to years (although it may be abrupt after head trauma or vascular insult). Individuals with dementia usually have a stable presentation over brief periods of time, although they may also have nocturnal worsening of symptoms ("sundowning"). Memory impairment is often greatest for short-term memory. Recall of names is frequently impaired, as is recognition

TABLE 8-4 Specific Diseases Associated with Dementia	
Disease	**Description**
Alzheimer's	Most common cause of dementia, accounts for greater than 50% of all cases. Risk factors are familial, Down syndrome, prior head trauma, increasing age. Clinically, it is a diagnosis of exclusion. Post-mortem pathology reveals cortical atrophy, neurofibrillary tangles, amyloid plaques, granulovacuolar degeneration, loss of basal forebrain cholinergic nuclei. Course is progressive, death occurs 8 to 10 years after onset.
Vascular	Second most common cause of dementia. Risk factors are cardiovascular and cerebrovascular disease. Neuroimaging reveals multiple areas of neuronal damage. Neurological exam reveals focal findings. Course can be rapid onset or more slowly progressive. Deficits are not reversible, but progress can be halted with appropriate treatment of vascular disease.
HIV	Limited to those cases caused by direct action of HIV on the brain; associated illnesses, such as meningitis, lymphoma, toxoplasmosis producing dementia are categorized under dementia due to general medical conditions. Primarily affects white matter and cortex.
Head trauma	Most common among young males. Extent of dementia is determined by degree of brain damage. Deficits are stable unless there is repeated head trauma.
Parkinson's	Occurs in 20% to 60% of individuals with Parkinson's disease. The most likely pathological finding on autopsy is Lewy body disease. Bradyphrenia (slowed thinking) is common. Some individuals also have pathology at autopsy consistent with Alzheimer's dementia.
Huntington's	Risk factors are familial, autosomal dominant on chromosome 4. Onset commonly in mid 30s. Emotional lability is prominent. Caudate atrophy is present on autopsy.
Pick's	Onset at age 50 to 60. Frontal and temporal atrophy are prominent on neuroimaging. The dementia responds poorly to psychotropic medicine.
Creutzfeldt–Jakob	Familial in 10% of cases. Onset age 40 to 60. Prion is thought to be agent of transmission. Clinical triad of dementia, myoclonus, and abnormal EEG. Rapidly progressive. Spongiform encephalopathy is present at autopsy.

of familiar objects. Executive functions of organization and planning may be lost. Paranoia, hallucinations, and delusions are often present. Eventually, individuals with dementia may become mute, incontinent, and bedridden.

Differential Diagnosis

Dementia should be differentiated from delirium. In addition, dementia should be differentiated from those developmental disorders (such as mental retardation) with impaired cognition. Individuals with major depression and psychosis can appear to suffer dementia; they warrant a diagnosis of dementia only if their cognitive deficits cannot be fully attributed to the primary psychiatric illness.

A critical component of differential diagnosis in dementia is to distinguish pseudodementia associated with depression. Although there are many precise criteria for separating the two disorders, neuropsychological testing may be needed to make an accurate diagnosis. In pseudodementia, mood symptoms are prominent and patients may complain extensively of memory impairment. They characteristically give "I don't know" answers to mental status examination queries but may answer correctly if pressed. Memory is intact with rehearsal in pseudodementia, but not in dementia.

MANAGEMENT

Dementia from reversible, or treatable, causes should be managed first by treating the underlying cause of the dementia; rehabilitation may be required for residual deficits. Reversible (or partially reversible) causes of dementia include normal pressure hydrocephalus; neurosyphilis; HIV infection; and thiamine, folate, vitamin B_{12}, and niacin deficiencies. Vascular dementias may not be reversible, but their progress can be halted in some cases. Nonreversible dementias are usually managed by placing the patient in a safe environment and by medications targeted at associated symptoms. There are four acetylcholinesterase inhibitor medications (tacrine, rivastigmine, donepezil, and galantamine) currently approved for the treatment of Alzheimer's dementia. Tacrine has the highest rate of hepatotoxicity. The acetylcholinesterase inhibitors improve cognitive function and global function. High-potency antipsychotics (in low doses) are used when agitation, paranoia, and hallucinations are present. Atypical antipsychotic medications are often used as well but appear to

increase the risk of stroke and other forms of mortality in elderly individuals. Low-dose benzodiazepines and trazodone are often used for anxiety, agitation, or insomnia. However, both benzodiazepines and trazodone may increase the risk of falls and should be used sparingly.

🔑 8-2 KEY POINTS

1. Dementia is a disorder of memory impairment coupled with other cognitive defects.
2. Dementia has a gradual onset and progressive course.
3. Dementia may be caused by a variety of illnesses.
4. Dementia predisposes to delirium.

AMNESTIC DISORDERS

Amnestic disorders are isolated disturbances of memory without impairment of other cognitive functions. They may be due to a general medical condition or may be substance related.

ETIOLOGY

Amnestic disorders are caused by general medical conditions or substance use. Common general medical conditions include head trauma, hypoxia, herpes simplex encephalitis, and posterior cerebral artery infarction. Amnestic disorders often are associated with damage of the mammillary bodies, fornix, and hippocampus. Bilateral damage to these structures produces the most severe deficits. Amnestic disorders due to substance-related causes may be the result of substance abuse, use of prescribed or over-the-counter medications, or accidental exposure to toxins. Alcohol abuse is a leading cause of substance-related amnestic disorder. Persistent alcohol use may lead to thiamine deficiency and induce Wernicke–Korsakoff's syndrome. If properly treated, the acute symptoms of ataxia, abnormal eye movements, and confusion may resolve, leaving a residual amnestic disorder called Korsakoff psychosis (alcohol-induced persistent amnestic disorder).

EPIDEMIOLOGY

Individuals affected by a general medical condition or alcoholism are at risk for amnestic disorders.

CLINICAL MANIFESTATIONS

History and Mental Status Examination

Amnestic disorders present as **deficits in memory**, either in the inability to recall previously learned information or the inability to retain new information. The cognitive defect must be limited to memory alone; if additional cognitive defects are present, a diagnosis of dementia or delirium should be considered. In addition to defect in memory, there must be an identifiable cause for the amnestic disorder (i.e., the presence of a general medical condition or substance use).

Differential Diagnosis

Delirium and dementia are the major differential diagnostic considerations. Amnestic disorders are distinguished from dissociative disorders on the basis of etiology. By definition, amnestic disorders are due to a general medical condition or substance.

MANAGEMENT

The general medical condition is treated whenever possible to prevent further neurologic damage; in the case of a substance-related amnestic disorder, avoiding re-exposure to the substance responsible for the amnestic disorder is critical. Pharmacotherapy may be directed at treating associated anxiety or mood difficulties. Patients should be placed in a safe, structured environment with frequent memory cues.

🔑 8-3 KEY POINTS

1. Amnestic disorders are disorders in memory alone.
2. The disorders are caused by identifiable precipitants.
3. Amnestic disorders are reversible in some cases.

References

Cummings JL. Alzheimer's disease. *N Engl J Med.* 2004 Jul 1;351(1):56–67.

de Rooij SE, Schuurmans MJ, van der Mast RC, et al. Clinical subtypes of delirium and their relevance for daily clinical practice: a systematic review. *Int J Geriatr Psychiatry.* 2005 Jul;20(7): 609–615.

Pandharipande P, Jackson J, Ely EW. Delirium: acute cognitive dysfunction in the critically ill. *Curr Opin Crit Care.* 2005 Aug;11(4):360–368.

Pietrzik C, Behl C. Concepts for the treatment of Alzheimer's disease: molecular mechanisms and clinical application. *Int J Exp Pathol.* 2005 Jun;86(3):173–185.

Miscellaneous Disorders

Miscellaneous disorders do not refer to any official *Diagnostic and Statistical Manual of Mental Disorders*, 4th edition (DSM-IV) classification but rather to psychiatric diagnoses not covered elsewhere in this book. Generally, these diagnoses are either less common, less understood, or less frequently the focus of psychiatric practice than the disorders previously covered. Although many of these disorders are not uncommon, they seldom come to psychiatric attention for a variety of reasons (e.g., they may be treated by other medical specialists, patients may not mention them, or they may not be detected adequately). Table 9-1 lists the categories of disorders discussed in this chapter.

DISSOCIATIVE DISORDERS

Dissociative disorders are characterized by disturbances in the integration of mental functions. These disturbances are manifested by loss of memory for personal information or identity, division of consciousness and personality into separate parts, and altered perception of the environment or sense of reality. Table 9-2 lists DSM-IV defined dissociative disorders.

DISSOCIATIVE AMNESIA

In dissociative amnesia, an individual develops a temporary inability to recall important personal information. The amnesia is more extensive than forgetfulness and is not caused by another medical or psychiatric condition (e.g., head trauma). The inability to recall information may take several forms. In **localized amnesia**, information is lost for a specific time period (e.g., a time associated with trauma). In **selective amnesia**, some information during a given time period is retained but other information is lost. In **generalized amnesia**, personal information is lost for the entire life span. In **continuous amnesia**, there is an inability to recall information from a single point in time to the present. In **systematized amnesia**, particular categories of information are lost to retrieval.

Dissociative amnesia is more common in people exposed to trauma, for example, those exposed to battle or natural disaster.

DISSOCIATIVE FUGUE

Dissociative fugue is an amnestic disorder characterized by an individual's sudden unexplained travel away from home, coupled with amnesia for his or her identity. In this condition, patients do not appear mentally ill or otherwise impaired in any other mental function, including memory. In fact, patients are quite capable of negotiating the complexities of travel and interaction with others. In rare cases, an individual will establish a completely new identity in the new home. Dissociative fugue is typically precipitated by a severe trauma or stressor and eventually remits without treatment.

DISSOCIATIVE IDENTITY DISORDER

Dissociative identity disorder (formerly called multiple personality disorder) is a controversial diagnosis in psychiatry. The diagnosis of dissociative identity disorder requires the presence of two or more separate personalities (alters) that recurrently take control of an individual's behavior. Individuals with this disorder often have amnesia for important personal information (also known as "losing time"). The various personalities (the average number by available surveys is seven distinct personalities) may be unaware of each other's existence and thus may be quite confused as to how they arrived

■ **TABLE 9-1** Miscellaneous Disorders
Dissociative disorders
Somatoform disorders
Adjustment disorders
Sexual and gender identity disorders
Sleep disorders
Factitious disorders/malingering

at certain places or why they cannot recall personal events. At other times, one or more personalities may be aware of the others, a condition known as coconsciousness. Some personalities may display conversion symptoms or self-mutilating behavior. The alters may be of varying ages and different genders and demeanors.

Dissociative identity disorder is most common in females and has a chronic course. Individuals with dissociative identity disorder are highly suggestible and easily hypnotized. Most report a childhood history of severe physical or sexual abuse. Satanic or cult abuse reports are also common. In many cases, these reports of abuse cannot be verified, leading many clinicians to believe that individuals with dissociative identity disorder may suffer from memories of events that did not occur. Whether these memories are true or false, they cause a great deal of suffering.

Disagreement over the very nature of dissociative identity disorder has led to divergent treatment opinions.

Some clinicians believe that ignoring the different personalities will cause them to recede, based on the notion that the easy suggestibility of these patients will lead to reinforcement of alters if they are discussed. Others believe that long-term psychotherapy, exploring the various personalities and integrating them into a whole person, is the treatment of choice.

Overall, the currently available scientifically verifiable evidence does not support the diagnosis of dissociative identity disorder as a unique diagnosis; further, there is little support for the association between trauma and symptoms of this condition.

DEPERSONALIZATION DISORDER

Depersonalization disorder is characterized by "persistent or recurrent experiences of feeling detached from and as if one is an outside observer of one's mental processes or body" (DSM-IV). Individuals with this disorder may complain of a sense of detachment, of feeling mechanical or automated, and of absence of affect or sensation. Individuals with depersonalization disorder are easily hypnotized and prone to dissociate.

SOMATOFORM DISORDERS

Somatoform disorders are characterized by the presence of physical signs or symptoms without medical cause. In addition, they are *not* willfully produced by the individual. Namely, in contradistinction to factitious disorder and malingering, the symptoms of somatoform disorders are assumed to be **subconscious** in origin. The somatoform disorders are listed and defined in Table 9-3.

SOMATIZATION DISORDER

Somatization disorder is diagnosed when an individual has multiple medical complaints that are not the result of medical illness. The specific DSM-IV criteria are narrow and specific, requiring

- Pain in four different body sites or involving four different body functions;
- Two gastrointestinal symptoms (other than pain);
- One sexual symptom (other than pain); and
- One pseudoneurologic symptom (other than pain).

In addition, some symptoms must have begun before age 30 and persisted for several years. Individuals with

■ **TABLE 9-2** Dissociative Disorders	
Dissociative amnesia	Temporary inability to recall important personal information; more serious than simple forgetfulness
Dissociative fugue	Amnesia for one's identity coupled with sudden unexplained travel away from home
Dissociative identity disorder	Presence of two or more separate personalities that recurrently take control of a person's behavior
Depersonalization disorder	Pervasive sense of being detached from or being outside of one's body

■ TABLE 9-3 Somatoform Disorders

Somatization disorder	Chronic multiple medical complaints that include pain, gastrointestinal disturbance, sexual symptoms, and pseudoneurologic symptoms that are not due to a medical illness
Undifferentiated somatoform disorder	A less severe form of somatization disorder; involves fewer complaints and briefer course
Conversion disorder	Complaints involving sensory (such as numbness) and voluntary motor (such as paralysis) function that are not due to neurologic dysfunction
Pain disorder	Pain is the major complaint; if medical causes are present, psychological factors have a major role in mediating the expression and impact of pain
Hypochondriasis	Preoccupation with having a serious disease based on a misinterpretation of bodily function and sensation
Body dysmorphic disorder	Excessive concern with a perceived defect in appearance

Adapted from DSM-IV.

somatization disorder often have a history of complex medical and surgical treatments that may actually lead to iatrogenic complications of treatment. Patients with somatoform disorder frequently have multiple physicians, make frequent office and hospital visits, and may seek disability because of their conviction that they are severely and chronically medically ill.

This disorder is more common in females (approximately 80% of cases), and its incidence is increased in first-degree relatives of those with somatization disorder. Familial and genetic studies have also shown that male relatives of individuals with somatization disorder have an increased incidence of antisocial personality disorder (ASP) and substance abuse. Adoption studies suggest genetic influences in this disorder.

Various theories have been proposed to explain this disorder. Early psychoanalytic work focused on repressed instincts as causative; more modern theorists propose that somatization symptoms may represent a means of nonverbal interpersonal communication. Biologic findings have revealed abnormal cortical function in some individuals with this disorder. Overall, the disorder appears to be best explained using an integrated bio-psycho-social approach grounded in cognitive interpretations and learning theory.

Cognitive-behavioral therapy is the most effective treatment for somatization disorder. Antidepressant medications are also helpful in patients with or without comorbid depressive symptoms. Additional strategies for treating somatization include regular, structured visits by a single physician with the goal of avoiding excessive or invasive diagnostic workups and visits by the patient to other physicians or emergency wards.

ADJUSTMENT DISORDERS

According to DSM-IV, adjustment disorders are symptoms (changes in emotional state or behaviors) that arise in response to an identified psychosocial stressor that is out of proportion to what is expected in usual human experience. Adjustment disorder is not diagnosed if the symptoms occurred in response to a psychosocial stressor so severe that an individual meets criteria for another axis I disorder (e.g., major depression). Symptoms in response to bereavement do not meet criteria for the diagnosis of adjustment disorder. Adjustment disorders occur within 3 months of the identified stressor and usually resolve within 6 months, unless the stressor becomes chronic.

SEXUAL AND GENDER IDENTITY DISORDERS

The DSM-IV classifies these disorders into sexual dysfunctions, paraphilia, and gender identity disorders.

SEXUAL DYSFUNCTIONS

Sexual dysfunctions are sexual disorders associated with alterations in the sexual response cycle (Table 9-4) or with pain associated with sexual activity. The specific sexual dysfunctions are defined in Table 9-5.

■ TABLE 9-4 Sexual Response Cycle	
Desire	Initial stage of sexual response; consists of sexual fantasies and the urge to have sex
Excitement	Consists of physiologic arousal and feeling of sexual pleasure
Orgasm	Peaking sexual pleasure; usually associated with ejaculation in men
Resolution	Physiologic relaxation associated with sense of well-being; in men, there is usually a refractory period for further excitement and orgasm

PARAPHILIAS

Paraphilias include sexual disorders related to culturally unusual sexual activity (Table 9-6). A key criterion for the diagnosis of a paraphilia (as in all psychiatric disorders) is that the disorder must cause an individual to experience significant distress or impairment in social or occupational functioning. In other words, an individual with unusual sexual practices who does not suffer significant distress or impairment would not be diagnosed with a psychiatric illness.

GENDER IDENTITY DISORDER

Gender identity disorder remains a controversial diagnosis in psychiatry. Individuals with this disorder experience distress and interpersonal impairment as a result of their desire to be a member of the opposite sex. Criteria for the diagnosis require a pervasive cross-gender identification and persistent discomfort with one's assigned sex. In addition, the diagnosis is made only in those individuals who do not have an intersex condition (e.g., ambiguous genitalia). Children with this disorder may engage in gender-atypical play; adults may assume the societal role, dress, and behavior associated with the opposite sex. In addition, patients with gender identity disorder may seek sex reassignment surgery and hormonal supplements. Individuals with gender identity disorder appear to have the same range of sexual orientations as do persons without this disorder.

■ TABLE 9-5 Specific Sexual Dysfunctions		
Sexual desire disorders	Hypoactive sexual desire disorder	Sexual fantasy and desire for sex very low or absent
	Sexual aversion disorder	Aversion to genital sexual contact with another person
Sexual arousal disorders	Female sexual arousal disorder	Inadequate vaginal lubrication and inadequate engorgement of external genitalia
Orgasmic disorders	Male erectile disorder	Inability to attain or maintain an erection
	Female orgasmic disorder	Orgasm is absent or delayed; sexual excitement phase is normal
	Male orgasmic disorder	Orgasm is absent or delayed; sexual excitement phase is normal
	Premature ejaculation	Orgasm and ejaculation occur early and with minimal stimulation
Sexual pain disorders	Dyspareunia	Genital pain in association with sexual intercourse
	Vaginismus	Involuntary contraction of external vaginal musculature as a result of attempted penetration
Sexual dysfunction due to a general medical condition		
Substance-induced sexual dysfunction		

■ TABLE 9-6 Paraphilias

Exhibitionism	Sexual excitement is derived from exposing one's genitals to a stranger.
Fetishism	Nonliving objects are the focus of intense sexual arousal in fantasy or behavior.
Frotteurism	Sexual excitement is derived by rubbing one's genitals against or by sexually touching a nonconsenting stranger.
Pedophilia	Sexual excitement is derived from fantasy or behavior involving sex with prepubescent children.
Sexual masochism	Sexual excitement is derived from fantasy or behavior involving being the recipient of humiliation, bondage, or pain.
Sexual sadism	Sexual excitement is derived from fantasy or behavior involving inflicting suffering/humiliation on another.
Transvestic fetishism	Sexual excitement (in heterosexual men) is derived from fantasy or behavior involving wearing women's clothing.
Voyeurism	Sexual excitement is derived from fantasy or behavior involving the observation of unsuspecting individuals undressing, naked, or having sex.

SLEEP DISORDERS

Sleep disorders are illnesses related to alterations in the sleep–wake cycle (Table 9-7) and often have effects on mood, cognitive, somatic, and general performance. Table 9-8 outlines the DSM-IV classification of sleep disorders. Sleep disorders are categorized into primary and secondary sleep disorders. Primary sleep disorders are those disorders occurring as a direct result of disturbances in the sleep–wake cycle. They are divided into two categories: dyssomnias and parasomnias. Secondary sleep disorders are a consequence of other mental disorders (e.g., depression) due to general medical conditions (e.g., somatic pain) or substance use (e.g., caffeine).

■ TABLE 9-7 Sleep Stages

Non-rapid eye movement (NREM)		
	Stage 0	Awake.
	Stage 1	Very light[a] sleep, transition from wakefulness to sleep. Drowsy.
	Stage 2	Medium depth of sleep, occupies about half the night in adults. Serves as a transition stage between rapid eye movement (REM) and delta sleep. EEG demonstrates sleep spindles and k-complexes.
		Slow wave sleep, composed of stages 3 and 4, occupies 10%–30% of total sleep.
	Delta	
	Stage 3	Consists of a moderate amount of delta wave activity; deeper sleep than stage 2.
	Stage 4	Increased delta wave activity over stage 3. Very deep stage of sleep.
REM		Dream sleep. EEG is active, mimicking that of the waking stage. Depth of sleep is greater than stage 2 but probably less than delta.

[a]Depth of sleep as used here is not a precise term but generally refers to ease of arousability (i.e., how hard would it be to awaken an individual from a particular stage). However, the ease of arousability is due in part to the type of stimulus used (e.g., noise versus touch).

■ TABLE 9-8 Sleep Disorders

Primary Sleep Disorders	Secondary Sleep Disorders
Dyssomnias	
Primary insomnia	Sleep disorder related to another mental disorder
Primary hypersomnia	
Narcolepsy	Sleep disorder due to a general medical condition
Breathing-related sleep disorder	Substance-induced sleep disorder
Circadian rhythm sleep disorder	
Parasomnias	
Nightmare disorder	
Sleep terror disorder	
Sleepwalking disorder	

DYSSOMNIAS

Dyssomnias are five primary sleep disorders consisting of disturbances in initiating and maintaining sleep, feeling rested or refreshed after sleep, or sleeping excessively.

Table 9-9 defines the DSM-IV determined key characteristics of each disorder.

Chronic Insomnia

Of the sleep disorders, none is more prevalent in psychiatry than insomnia either of primary origin or associated with other conditions such as anxiety, depression, or psychoactive substance use. Chronic insomnia is not an official DSM-IV category but is a clinical category arising from both primary and secondary insomnia and mixtures of the two. Insomnia can generally be considered chronic if it is of greater than 6 months duration. An estimated 15% of people have chronic insomnia. Factors increasing the risk for chronic insomnia include advancing age, psychiatric illness, medical illness, social stress (work, relationships, etc.), and female gender. The treatment of chronic insomnia remains a major challenge. Cognitive-behavioral therapy and relaxation therapy may be helpful. Modest effects have been noted for sleeping agents of various classes. Antidepressants may also have some effect but may also cause insomnia. There is a risk of benzodiazepine dependence from chronic use of benzodiazepines. Improved sleep hygiene, in the form of regular

■ TABLE 9-9 Primary Sleep Disorders

Dyssomnias	Primary insomnia	Difficulty falling asleep or staying asleep, or sleeping but feeling as if one has not rested during sleep.
	Primary hypersomnia	Excess sleepiness, either sleeping too long at one setting or persistent daytime sleepiness not relieved by napping.
	Narcolepsy	Sleep attacks during the daytime coupled with REM sleep intrusions or cataplexy (sudden, reversible bilateral loss of skeletal muscle tone). Daytime naps relieve sleepiness.
	Breathing-related sleep disorder	Abnormal breathing during sleep leads to sleep disruption and daytime sleepiness.
	Circadian rhythm sleep disorder	Sleep disturbance due to a mismatch between a person's intrinsic circadian rhythm and external sleep–wake demands.
Parasomnias	Nightmare disorder	Repeated episodes of scary dreams that wake a person from sleep, usually occur during *REM* sleep.
	Sleep terror disorder	Repeated episodes of apparent terror during sleep; individuals may sit up, scream, or cry out and appear extremely frightened. They do not usually awaken during the attack. Occurs during *delta* sleep.
	Sleepwalking disorder	Recurrent sleepwalking, often coupled with other complex motor activity.

sleep–wake cycles, avoidance of caffeine, and regular exercise may also prove beneficial.

PARASOMNIAS

Parasomnias are a triad of sleep disorders associated with complex behavioral events that occur during sleep or that arouse a person from sleep. The disorders are defined in Table 9-9.

FACTITIOUS DISORDERS

A factitious disorder is one in which an individual willfully produces signs or symptoms of a medical or psychiatric illness to assume the sick role and its associated gratifications. This should be differentiated from **somatoform disorders** (which are not willful) and **malingering**, which is simply lying about signs or symptoms to obtain gains different from those obtained by assuming the sick role (e.g., to avoid the military or for monetary gain).

9-1 KEY POINTS

1. Somatoform disorders include somatization disorder, undifferentiated somatoform disorder, conversion disorder, pain disorder, hypochondriasis, and body dysmorphic disorder.
2. The symptoms of somatization disorders are subconscious in origin.
3. Treatment of somatization disorder includes cognitive-behavioral therapy, antidepressants, and single-physician structured treatment.
4. Paraphilias are sexual behaviors or interests that are considered culturally unusual.
5. The primary sleep disorders include the dyssomnias and the parasomnias.
6. Sexual dysfunctions are categorized according to the phase of the sexual response cycle during which they occur or to the presence of pain.
7. Factitious disorder is characterized by the willful production of symptoms of illness in order to assume the sick role.

References

Buscemi N, Vandermeer B, Friesen C, et al. Manifestations and management of chronic insomnia in adults. *Evid Rep Technol Assess (Summ)*. 2005 Jun;(125):1–10.

Mai F. Somatization disorder: a practical review. *Can J Psychiatry*. 2004 Oct;49(10):652–662.

Piper A, Merskey H. The persistence of folly: a critical examination of dissociative identity disorder. Part I. The excesses of an improbable concept. *Can J Psychiatry*. 2004 Sep;49(9):592–600.

SUICIDE ATTEMPTS

EPIDEMIOLOGY

Suicide is the eighth leading cause of death in the United States. Approximately 75 people commit suicide each day in the United States (25,000 per year). Many more people attempt suicide. The overall suicide rate has remained stable in the United States during the past 15 years. Although the rate of suicide in teenagers aged 15 to 19 is low compared with the general adult population, the rate of teen suicide has risen dramatically in the last 50 years.

RISK FACTORS

Studies have demonstrated that the overwhelming majority of people who commit suicide have a mental illness (most often a mood disorder or chronic alcoholism). The first-degree relatives of people who have committed suicide are at a much higher risk of committing suicide themselves. Gay and lesbian youth have two to three times the rate of attempted suicide compared to heterosexual adolescents. Suicide risk increases with age. In men, suicides peak after age 45; in women, most suicides occur after age 55. Elderly individuals account for 25% of the suicides, although they represent only 10% of the population. Overall, men are more successful at completing suicide, perhaps because of their more lethal methods (shooting, hanging, jumping); women often overdose or attempt drowning. Married people have a lower risk of suicide than singles. Suicide is more common among higher social classes, whites, and certain professional groups (physicians, dentists, musicians, law enforcement officers, lawyers, and insurance agents). Biologic risk factors include low levels of

5-hydroxyindoleacetic acid in the cerebrospinal fluid of patients who have committed suicide by violent means. Among psychological risk factors, hopelessness has been shown to be one of the most reliable indicators of long-term suicide risk.

Recent evidence suggests that suicidal risk may increase in children and adolescents who initiate treatment with antidepressant medication (for depression or other psychiatric conditions). The details of the association between antidepressant medication treatment and child and adolescent suicidality are unknown. Antidepressant medication prescribing information in the United States now contains a black box warning cautioning providers to assess carefully the risks and benefits of antidepressant treatment in children and adolescents. Providers should also warn patients and their families that suicidal thinking may increase with antidepressant medication treatment, especially during the first few months of treatment. Because antidepressants may also transiently increase suicidality in adults as well, adult patients should also be cautioned regarding this possibility. Periods of initiating, tapering, or adjusting the dosage of an antidepressant medication may increase the risk of worsening depression or suicidality—these periods warrant extra scrutiny by patients, families, and caregivers.

CLINICAL MANIFESTATIONS

History and Mental Status Examination

Most often, a suicide attempt is self-evident at presentation, either because the patient or family indicates that such an event has occurred or because there is an acute medical or surgical emergency (i.e., overdose or wrist laceration). It is important always to obtain further details from the patient and any witnesses to provide a full history of the antecedents and the suicidal act. Occasionally, a patient will present to a physician in a more subtle way, with nonspecific complaints. Patients may also overtly deny suicidal intent, even when prior statements to intimates or caregivers indicate clear suicidal thinking or planning. Careful inquiry may reveal that the patient has taken an overdose of a medication with delayed lethality (such as acetaminophen).

Patients who have attempted suicide deserve thorough psychiatric evaluation. Psychiatric history and mental status examination should explicitly address depressive symptoms, such as suicidal thoughts, intent, and plans. The details of the suicide attempt are critical to understanding the risk of a future suicide. Patients who carefully plan the attempt, use particularly violent means, and isolate themselves so as not to be found alive are at particularly high risk of future suicide completion.

Differential Diagnosis

Patients who attempt suicide most commonly suffer from depression, schizophrenia, alcoholism, or personality disorders (or comorbidities of the above). However, patients who do not meet criteria for any of these disorders can and do attempt or commit suicide, especially if they have any of the risk factors (e.g., hopelessness).

MANAGEMENT

Suicidal ideation should always be taken seriously. Suicidal patients often are fraught with ambivalence over whether to live or die, and intervention and effective treatment can be lifesaving. Most actively suicidal patients require hospitalization on a locked unit for their own safety. Potentially lethal items should be held securely by nursing staff, and the patient should be observed carefully for the risk of elopement. Treatment of the underlying disorder or distress derives from accurate diagnosis—antidepressants or electroconvulsive therapy (ECT) for depression; antipsychotics and/or mood stabilizers for bipolar disorder, psychotic depression, or schizophrenia.

Patients at lower risk of suicide can often be managed as outpatients if close follow-up is available, family members are supportive, and a treatment alliance exists. Frequent meetings with treatment providers, eliminating the means of suicide (firearms, potentially toxic prescription pills), and enlisting spouses, partners, or other family members are essential elements of outpatient treatment.

Surprisingly, there is little solid empirical evidence to guide clinical intervention targeted at preventing suicide. While it seems clear that treating an underlying psychiatric condition might reduce the suicide risk associated with that condition, clear data are not yet available regarding the particular efficacy of a given medication or class in this regard. Psychosocial interventions targeted at preventing suicide do not have strong research support. Until additional evidence-based findings emerge, the standard of care for suicidal individuals remains hospitalization or other secure treatment alternative coupled to treatment of associated psychiatric conditions.

SPOUSAL ABUSE

Abuse between spouses or partners can take several forms: physical, sexual, and emotional. Physical abuse or battering is most often perpetrated by a male on a female partner, but women do batter men and abuse also occurs in same-sex relationships.

EPIDEMIOLOGY

Spousal abuse is estimated to occur in 2 to 12 million US households. Some studies estimate that nearly one third of all women have been beaten by their husband at least once during their marriage. Many battered women are eventually murdered by their spouses or boyfriends. According to the U.S. Department of Justice, 37% of women treated in emergency rooms for violent injuries were hurt by a current or former partner. Of women murdered by an intimate partner, 44% visited an emergency room in the 2 years prior to their deaths.

RISK FACTORS

There is a strong association between alcohol abuse and domestic violence. More than 50% of abusers, and many of the abused, have a history of alcohol or other drug abuse. As children, most abusers lived in violent homes where they either witnessed or were themselves victims of battering. The victims of abuse, more often than not, are also products of violent homes. Pregnant women are at elevated risk for spousal abuse, often directed at their abdomens.

CLINICAL MANIFESTATIONS

History and Physical and Mental Status Examination

Many victims of abuse are reluctant to report abusive episodes because they fear retaliation, believe they are deserving of abuse, or do not believe that help will be effective. Victims of abuse are often mistreated in ways that prevent them from escaping the abusive relationship. They are intimidated, maligned, coerced, and isolated by the abuser. Attempts to leave an abusive relationship may be thwarted by financial concerns, the welfare of children, fear of being alone, or the threat of further battering.

Patients may present in the company of their abuser for the treatment of "accidental" lacerations, contusions, fractures, or more severe trauma. Unless the patient is asked tactfully in the absence of the abuser, he or she is unlikely to reveal the true cause of injuries.

Physical examination should include examination of the skin for contusions (especially of the face and breasts) and a genital examination. The mental status examination should take into account the appropriateness of the patient's and partner's reactions to the "accident."

MANAGEMENT

The goal of treatment is to end the violence (i.e., both partners must agree to treatment) or to enable the victim to leave the relationship. Either option is difficult to achieve. Social agencies must be enlisted to aid in child protection and custody if the latter option is chosen.

Patients who refuse help should be told what emergency services are available and how to access them. Unfortunately, women are most at risk for serious injury or homicide when they attempt to leave the abusive relationship.

ELDER ABUSE

Approximately 10% of those older than age 65 are abused. Victims usually live with their assailants, who are often their children. Mistreatment includes abuse and neglect and takes physical, psychological, financial, and material forms. The abuser may withhold food, clothing, or other necessities or beat, sexually molest, or emotionally abuse the victim.

As with spousal abuse, the elder person is often reluctant to reveal the abuse. Clinicians should be alert to the signs of abuse. Treatment involves appropriate medical and psychiatric services and social and legal services. Some states mandate reporting of elder abuse.

BEREAVEMENT

Bereavement occurs following the death of a loved one. The DSM-IV criteria limit normal bereavement to a 2-month period following the loss of a loved one. The symptoms of bereavement, such as sad mood, trouble sleeping, loss of appetite, and ruminating on the loss of the loved one, mimic to some degree those of major depression. However, when symptoms of major depression predominate, or when the following symptoms occur, a diagnosis of major depression should be considered. Symptoms suggesting major depression include:

1. Increased guilt (not associated with behavior or actions related to the death of the loved one);
2. Suicidal thinking or thoughts of death (other than feeling that one has a desire to join the loved one in death);
3. Excess worthlessness;
4. Psychomotor retardation;
5. Severe impairment in ability to function;
6. Auditory or visual hallucinations (other than hearing the voice or image of the deceased, which is considered a normal component of bereavement).

Treatment for uncomplicated bereavement is diverse and there is not sufficient evidence available to suggest that one form of therapeutic intervention is reliably superior to another. In bereaved individuals with depression, antidepressant medication is indicated.

10-1 KEY POINTS

1. Suicide is a fatal complication of many psychiatric disorders.
2. Hopelessness is a risk factor for attempting suicide.
3. Antidepressants may transiently increase the risk of suicide.
4. About one third of females suffer spousal abuse.
5. About 10% of individuals over age 65 suffer elder abuse.
6. Normal bereavement lasts up to 2 months.
7. Antidepressant medications are indicated for the treatment of depression in bereaved individuals.

References

Forte AL, Hill M, Pazder R, et al. Bereavement care interventions: a systematic review. *BMC Palliat Care*. 2004 Jul 26;3(1):3.

Hawton K, James A. Suicide and deliberate self harm in young people. *Br Med J*. 2005 Apr 16;330(7496):891–894. Review.

Licinio J, Wong ML. Depression, antidepressants and suicidality: a critical appraisal. *Nat Rev Drug Discov*. 2005 Feb;4(2):165–171. Review.

Soomro GM. Deliberate self harm (and attempted suicide).*Clin Evid*. 2005 Jun;(13):1200–1211.

Antipsychotics

Antipsychotic medications are used commonly in medical and psychiatric practice. As a class, antipsychotics have in common their blockade of dopamine receptors and their potential for serious side effects if used inappropriately or without careful monitoring. The most commonly prescribed typical and atypical antipsychotics are listed in Tables 11-1 and 11-2. Their relative potencies, relative side-effect profiles, and major adverse reactions also are described. **Typical antipsychotics** (also called neuroleptics for their tendency to cause movement disorders) are generally equally effective, although they differ in side-effect profiles and potencies. **Atypical antipsychotics** (e.g., risperidone and clozapine) have fewer extrapyramidal side effects at therapeutic doses compared to typical antipsychotics. Clozapine (and perhaps other atypical antipsychotics) are more effective than typical antipsychotics for the treatment of refractory psychotic disorders.

INDICATIONS

Antipsychotics generally are effective in treating positive psychotic symptoms (e.g., hallucinations, bizarre behavior, delusions) regardless of diagnostic category (Table 11-3). For example, hallucinations in schizophrenia, in Alzheimer's disease, or secondary to cerebral toxicity or injury all respond to antipsychotic medications. Typical antipsychotics are thought to be less effective than atypical antipsychotics in treating negative psychotic symptoms (e.g., amotivation, akinesia, affective blunting, social withdrawal). In addition to their role in treating psychotic symptoms, antipsychotics are used to treat bipolar disorder (for acute mania and bipolar disorder maintenance), some forms of nonpsychotic behavioral dyscontrol (e.g., organic brain syndromes, Alzheimer's disease, mental retardation),

delirium, Tourette's syndrome, posttraumatic stress disorder symptoms, and transient psychotic symptoms as they appear in patients with personality disorder.

MECHANISM OF ACTION

The most prominent theory on the mechanism of action of antipsychotics is the **dopamine hypothesis** of schizophrenia. This hypothesis purports that dopaminergic hyperactivity leads to psychosis (Figure 11-1). Evidence supporting a role for hyperdopaminergic states in schizophrenia (and presumably other psychotic conditions) is as follows: antipsychotic potency of traditional antipsychotics correlates highly with their potency of dopamine receptor blockade, individuals with schizophrenia have an increased number of brain dopamine receptors, and dopamine agonist drugs (e.g., amphetamine) can induce or exacerbate existing psychosis.

The action mechanism of antipsychotics is often much broader than simple dopamine blockade, which accounts for the numerous side effects and the finding that their action in the brain is not well correlated with regions thought to give rise to psychotic symptoms. In addition, newer atypical antipsychotic medications have prominent serotonin (5-hydroxytryptamine-2 [$5HT_2$]) receptor activity. It is unclear whether this serotonin activity imparts antipsychotic efficacy, but the activity may affect mood and anxiety symptoms in patients with psychotic disorders and helps prevent extrapyramidal side effects.

Typical Antipsychotics (Dopamine Antagonists)

The antipsychotic potency of typical antipsychotics (and risperidone) correlates with their affinity for the D_2 receptor. Figure 11-2 is a schematic diagram of the proposed brain pathways affected by typical

TABLE 11-1 Typical Antipsychotics

Drug	Therapeutic Dosage Range[a]	Potency[b]	Sedative	Hypotensive	Anticholinergic	EPS
Typical antipsychotics (dopamine antagonists)						
Thioridazine (Mellaril)[c]	150–800 mg	100	High	High	High	Low
Chlorpromazine (Thorazine)	200–800 mg	100	High	High	Med	Low
Mesoridazine (Serentil)[c]	100–400 mg	50	Med	Med	Med	Med
Molindone (Moban)	15–225 mg	10	Med	Low	Med	High
Perphenazine (Trilafon)	8–32 mg	10	Low	Low	Low	Med
Loxapine (Loxitane, Daxolin)	60–100 mg	10	Med	Med	Med	High
Trifluoperazine (Stelazine)	5–20 mg	5	Med	Low	Low	High
Thiothixene (Navane)	5–30 mg	5	Low	Low	Low	High
Haloperidol (Haldol)	5–30 mg	2	Low	Low	Low	High
Fluphenazine (Prolixin)	2–60 mg	2	Med	Low	Low	High
Pimozide (Orap)	15–225 mg	1	Low	Low	Low	High

[a]Recommended initial starting dosages are lower than the therapeutic dosage. Dosages are generally lower for geriatric patients and for those who are taking interacting medications or have other medical problems. Adapted from Meltzer HY, Fatemi SH, Treatment of schizophrenia. In Schatzberg AF, Nemeroff CB, eds. *Textbook of psychopharmacology*, 2nd ed. Washington, DC: American Psychiatric Press, 1998.
[b]Potency is indicated as relative milligram dose equivalents (i.e., 100 mg of thioridazine is equivalent to 2 mg of haloperidol) and should not be confused with efficacy. All typical antipsychotics are thought to be equally efficacious.
[c]Due to fatal cardiac events, now approved only for refractory schizophrenia.
Based on Rosenbaum JF, et al. *Handbook of psychiatric drug therapy*. 5th ed. Philadelphia: Lippincott Williams & Wilkins, 2005.

antipsychotics. Dopamine-containing axons arising from brainstem nuclei (the ventral tegmental area and substantia nigra) project to the basal ganglia, frontal cortex, and limbic areas. Typical antipsychotics and risperidone strongly block D_2 receptors. Blockade of dopamine in the cortical and limbic areas results in reduction in psychotic symptoms, whereas blockade of dopamine in the basal ganglia produces extrapyramidal side effects. Although antipsychotics, especially lower potency medications, may have an initial sedative effect, their antipsychotic action is not immediate and takes several days to several weeks to peak.

Atypical Antipsychotics (Serotonin/Dopamine Antagonists)

At present, in the United States five atypical antipsychotics are marketed; others are likely to be available soon. Antipsychotics are classified as atypical when they produce fewer movement side effects than typical antipsychotics. In addition to dopamine receptor blockade, atypical antipsychotics block serotonin receptors of the $5HT_2$ subtype. Figure 11-3 depicts the similarities and differences of the serotonin and dopamine systems. Serotonin receptor blockade conveys some protection against extrapyramidal side effects and may impart antipsychotic efficacy. Risperidone is similar to typical neuroleptics in that it is a very potent blocker of the D_2 receptor. The mechanism of action of other atypical antipsychotics is more complex than simple D_2 receptor blockade.

TABLE 11-2 Atypical Antipsychotics

Drug	Therapeutic Daily Dosage Range
Aripiprazole (Abilify)	10–30 mg
Clozapine (Clozaril)	100–600 mg
Risperidone (Risperdal)	4–6 mg
Olanzapine (Zyprexa)	10–20 mg
Quetiapine (Seroquel)	400–800 mg
Ziprasidone (Geodon)	80–160 mg

■ TABLE 11-3 Indications for Antipsychotic Drugs

	Effective	Possibly Effective
Short-term use (<3 mo)	Exacerbations of schizophrenia	Brief use for episodes of severe dyscontrol or apparent psychosis in some personality disorders
	Acute mania	
	Depression with psychotics features (combined with antidepressant)	
	Other acute psychoses (e.g., schizophreniform psychoses)	
	Acute deliria and organic psychoses	
	Drug-induced psychoses due to hallucinogens and psychostimulants (not phencyclidine)	
	Nonpsychiatric uses: nausea and vomiting; movement disorders	
Long-term use (>3 mo)	Schizophrenia	Delusional disorders
	Tourette's syndrome	Childhood psychoses
	Treatment-resistant bipolar disorder	Posttraumatic stress disorder nightmares and flashbacks
	Huntington's disease and other movement disorders	
	Chronic psychoses related to neurologic disorders	

Modified and reproduced from Rosenbaum, JF, et al. *Handbook of psychiatric drug therapy.* 5th ed. Philadelphia: Lippincott Williams & Wilkins, 2005.

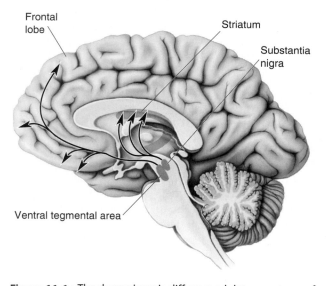

Figure 11-1 • The dopaminergic diffuse modulatory systems of the brain. The mesocorticolimbic dopamine system arises in the ventral tegmental area and has been implicated in the cause of schizophrenia. A second dopaminergic system arises from the substantia nigra and is involved in the control of voluntary movement by the striatum.
From Bear MF, Connors BW, Parasido, MA. *Neuroscience—exploring the brain,* 2nd ed. Philadelphia: Lippincott Williams & Wilkins. 2001.

CHOICE OF MEDICATION

Because all antipsychotics are considered efficacious, choice of medication should be based on prior patient or family member response, side-effect profile (patient tolerance), and available form (i.e., elixir or IM, or IM depot availability). At present, **clozapine** is the only medication clearly shown to be superior in patients for whom typical antipsychotics have failed. Fluphenazine and haloperidol are available in depot preparations, which are given intramuscularly every 2 to 4 weeks.

Olanzapine is also approved for use in acute bipolar mania and for the maintenance treatment of bipolar disorder in the United States. The intramuscular forms of olanzapine and ziprasidone are approved for agitation in schizophrenia. Atypical antipsychotics approved for bipolar disorder include olanzapine, quetiapine, risperidone, ziprasidone, and aripiprazole.

THERAPEUTIC MONITORING

Patients on antipsychotics should be monitored closely for adverse drug reactions. Particularly important are neurologic side effects such as akathisia (restlessness),

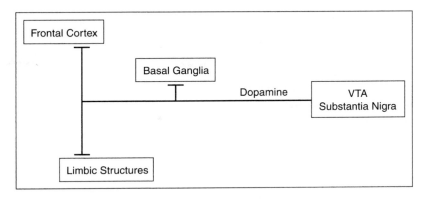

Figure 11-2 • Pathways affected by typical antipsychotics.

neuroleptic malignant syndrome (NMS), and extrapyramidal symptoms (EPS). Patients taking antipsychotics that lower seizure threshold should be carefully monitored for seizure activity. Individuals taking clozapine must have frequent white blood cell counts to monitor for the development of agranulocytosis. Clozapine must be discontinued immediately in patients demonstrating this potentially fatal reaction.

Blood levels have generally been of little use in monitoring antipsychotic efficacy but may be useful in assessing adherence. Haloperidol levels have some utility in patients who have side effects at low doses or who fail to respond to high doses. Clozapine levels are also frequently used to determine adherence and correlate efficacy with levels. Nonadherence is often the cause of apparent therapeutic failure.

The duration of therapy depends on the nature and severity of the patient's illness. Many disorders, such as schizophrenia, require maintenance antipsychotic therapy. Because of the serious sequela associated with long-term antipsychotic use, maintenance therapy should be used only after a careful risk-to-benefit analysis with the patient and involved family.

SIDE EFFECTS AND ADVERSE DRUG REACTIONS

Side effects of antipsychotics are a major consideration in physician prescribing. Patients who cannot bear the side effects of medications are nonadherent and suffer greater rates of relapse and recurrence. Certain side effects such as sedation can be useful to a patient with insomnia or severe agitation but can also limit functioning. A comparison of side-effect profiles for commonly used typical antipsychotics is provided in Table 11-1. Common side effects are described below. Further discussion of neurologic side effects is found in Chapter 16.

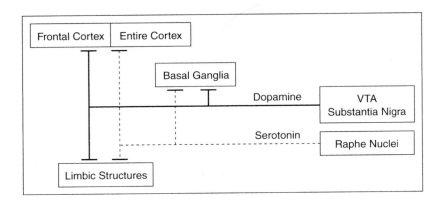

Figure 11-3 • Pathways affected by atypical antipsychotics.

Anticholinergic Side Effects

Low-potency antipsychotics have the greatest anticholinergic side effects such as dry mouth, constipation, urinary retention, and blurred vision. The anticholinergic properties, however, counter the EPS. In some cases, anticholinergic delirium may occur, especially in elderly individuals, those with organic brain syndromes, or patients on other anticholinergic agents.

Reduced Seizure Threshold

Low-potency typical antipsychotics and clozapine are associated with lowering seizure threshold. Seizures resulting from antipsychotic therapy are treated by changing medications, lowering the dose, or adding an antiseizure medication.

Hypotension

Orthostatic hypotension is particularly common with low-potency agents and risperidone. The hypotensive effect of antipsychotics is generally due to alpha-receptor blockade.

Agranulocytosis

Agranulocytosis has been associated most commonly with clozapine. Because of the potentially fatal nature of this adverse effect, clozapine distribution is regulated and requires a weekly complete blood count with differential to monitor for neutropenia.

Cardiac Side Effects

Ziprasidone, low-potency antipsychotics (particularly thioridazine and mesoridazine), and risperidone may cause QT prolongation (with risk of *torsade de pointes*). Nonspecific electrocardiographic changes may also occur with certain antipsychotic medications (particularly with clozapine and olanzapine). Clozapine can cause a myocarditis, which is rare, but most commonly occurs early in treatment.

Metabolic Effects

Although patients with psychotic disorders are known to have higher rates of obesity and diabetes mellitus independent of medication therapy, studies have indicated that atypical antipsychotic medications (particularly olanzapine and clozapine) are associated with high rates of weight gain, dyslipidemia, and may be associated with adult-onset diabetes. All patients taking these medications should have regular metabolic indices checked including lipid levels, fasting blood sugar, and body mass index.

Movement Disorders

Movement disorders such as dystonia, EPS, akathisia, NMS, and tardive dyskinesia may occur and are discussed further in Chapter 16.

Other Side Effects

Skin and ocular pigmentation are common side effects of neuroleptics, as is increased photosensitivity. Thioridazine can cause pigmentary retinopathy at high doses. Increased prolactin levels (and sequela) may also occur. Quetiapine may increase the risk of developing cataracts.

🔑 11-1 KEY POINTS

1. Antipsychotics are used to treat the psychotic symptoms of a wide range of disorders.
2. These drugs are probably equally effective but differ in potency (with the exception of clozapine).
3. Antipsychotics can have serious side effects.

References

Laruelle M, Frankle WG, Narendran R, et al. Mechanism of action of antipsychotic drugs: from dopamine D(2) receptor antagonism to glutamate NMDA facilitation. *Clin Ther.* 2005;27 suppl A:S16–24. Review.

Lieberman JA, Stroup TS, McEvoy JP, et al, and Clinical Antipsychotic Trials of Intervention Effectiveness (CATIE) Investigators. Effectiveness of antipsychotic drugs in patients with chronic schizophrenia. *N Engl J Med.* 2005 Sep 22;353(12):1209–1223.

Poulin MJ, Cortese L, Williams R, et al. Atypical antipsychotics in psychiatric practice: practical implications for clinical monitoring. *Can J Psychiatry.* 2005 Aug;50(9):555–562.

Chapter 12

Antidepressants, Electroconvulsive Therapy, and Phototherapy

Antidepressants are used commonly in medical and psychiatric practice. As a class, antidepressants have in common their ability to treat major depressive illness. Most antidepressants are also effective in the treatment of panic disorder and other anxiety disorders. Some antidepressants effectively treat obsessive–compulsive disorder (OCD) and a variety of other conditions (see indications below).

The most commonly prescribed antidepressants are listed in Table 12-1. Antidepressants are subdivided into groups based on structure or prominent functional activity: selective serotonin-reuptake inhibitors (SSRIs), tricyclic antidepressants (TCAs), monoamine oxidase inhibitors (MAOIs), and other antidepressant compounds with a variety of mechanisms of action.

Antidepressants are typically thought to act on either the serotonin or norepinephrine systems, or both (Figure 12-1). Choice of medications typically depends on diagnosis, history of response (in patient or relative), and the side-effect profile of the medication. Antidepressant effects are typically not seen until 2 to 4 weeks into treatment. Side effects must be carefully monitored, especially for TCAs and MAOIs.

INDICATIONS

Table 12-2 lists the indications for antidepressants. The main indication for antidepressant medications is major depressive disorder as defined by the *Diagnostic and Statistical Manual of Mental Disorders*, 4th edition (DSM-IV). Antidepressants are used in the treatment of all subtypes of depression, including depressed phase of bipolar disorder, psychotic depression (in combination with an antipsychotic medication), atypical depression, and seasonal depression (see Chapter 2). Antidepressants also are indicated for the prevention of recurrent depressive episodes.

Antidepressant medications may be effective in the treatment of patients with dysthymic disorder, especially when there are clear neurovegetative signs or a history of response to antidepressants.

Panic disorder with or without agoraphobia has been shown to respond to SSRIs, MAOIs, TCAs, and high-potency benzodiazepines (alprazolam and clonazepam).

OCD has been shown to respond to the serotonin-selective tricyclic clomipramine (Anafranil) and to SSRIs at high doses (e.g., fluoxetine at 60 to 80 mg per day). Obsessions tend to be more responsive to pharmacotherapy than compulsions. Symptoms of OCD respond more slowly than symptoms of major depression. Trials of 12 weeks or more are needed before a medication can be ruled a failure for a patient with OCD.

The binging and purging behavior of bulimia has been shown to respond to SSRIs, TCAs, and MAOIs in several open and controlled trials. Because SSRIs have the most benign side-effect profile of these medications, they are often the first-line psychopharmacologic treatment.

MECHANISMS OF ACTION

Antidepressants are thought to exert their effects at particular subsets of neuronal synapses throughout the brain. Their major interaction is with the monoamine neurotransmitter systems (dopamine, norepinephrine,

TABLE 12-1 Commonly Prescribed Antidepressants		
Drug (Brand Name)	**Usual Daily Dosage**[a]	**Extreme Daily Dosage**[a]
Selective serotonin reuptake inhibitors (SSRIs)		
Fluoxetine (Prozac)	20 mg	80 mg
Sertraline (Zoloft)	50–150 mg	300 mg
Paroxetine (Paxil)	20 mg	50 mg
Fluvoxamine (Luvox)	50–150 mg	300 mg
Citalopram (Celexa)	20–40 mg	60 mg
Escitalopram (Lexapro)	10 mg	30 mg
Serotonin-norepinephrine reuptake inhibitors (SNRIs)		
Venlafaxine (Effexor)	75–150 mg	450 mg
Duloxetine (Cymbalta)	40–60 mg	120 mg
Serotonin receptor agonists and antagonists		
Trazodone (Desyrel)	200–400 mg	600 mg
Nefazodone	200–450 mg	600 mg
Norepinephrine-dopamine reuptake inhibitors (NDRIs)		
Bupropion (Wellbutrin)	200–300 mg	450 mg
TCAs		
Nortriptyline (Pamelor)	75–100 mg	150 mg
Imipramine (Tofranil)	150–200 mg	300 mg
Desipramine (Norpramin)	150–200 mg	300 mg
Clomipramine (Anafranil)	150–200 mg	250 mg
MAOIs		
Tranylcypromine (Parnate)	30–50 mg	90 mg
Phenelzine (Nardil)	45–60 mg	90 mg
Isocarboxazid (Marplan)	30–50 mg	90 mg
Other antidepressants		
Mirtazapine (Remeron)	15–45 mg	60 mg

[a]Geriatric patients generally require lower doses.
Modified and reproduced from Rosenbaum JF, et al. *Handbook of psychiatric drug therapy.* 5th ed. Philadelphia: Lippincott Williams & Wilkins, 2005.

and serotonin). Dopamine, norepinephrine, and serotonin are released throughout the brain by neurons that originate in the ventral brainstem, locus ceruleus, and the raphe nuclei, respectively (Figures 12-1 and 12-2). These neurotransmitters interact with numerous receptor subtypes in the brain that are associated with the regulation of global state functions including

appetite, mood states, arousal, vigilance, attention, and sensory processing.

SSRIs act by binding to presynaptic serotonin reuptake proteins, thereby inhibiting reuptake and increasing the levels of serotonin in the synaptic cleft. TCAs act by blocking presynaptic reuptake of both serotonin and norepinephrine. MAOIs act by inhibiting the

Norepinephrine system

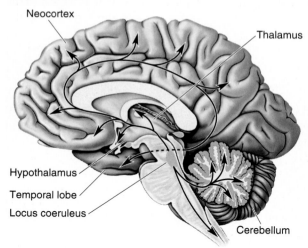

Figure 12-1 • The noradrenergic diffuse modulatory system arising from the locus coeruleus. The small cluster of locus coeruleus neurons project axons that innervate vast areas of the central nervous system, including the spinal cord, cerebellum, thalamus, and cerebral cortex.
From Bear MF, Connors BW, Parasido, MA. *Neuroscience—exploring the brain.* 2nd ed. Philadelphia: Lippincott Williams & Wilkins, 2001.

presynaptic enzyme (monoamine oxidase) that catabolizes norepinephrine, dopamine, and serotonin, thereby increasing the levels of these neurotransmitters presynaptically (Figure 12-3).

These immediate mechanisms of action are not sufficient to explain the delayed antidepressant effects (typically 2 to 4 weeks). Other, unknown mechanisms must play a role in the successful psychopharmacologic treatment of depression.

■ **TABLE 12-2** Indications for Antidepressants
Effective
Major depressive disorder and other unipolar depressive disorders
Bipolar depression
Panic disorder
Social phobia
Generalized anxiety disorder
Posttraumatic stress disorder
Obsessive–compulsive disorder (e.g., clomipramine and SSRIs)
Depression with psychotic features in combination with an antipsychotic drug
Bulimia nervosa
Neuropathic pain (tricyclic drugs and SNRIs)
Insomnia (e.g., trazodone, amitriptyline)
Enuresis (imipramine best studied)
Atypical depression (SSRIs or monoamine oxidase inhibitors)
Attention-deficit disorder with hyperactivity (e.g., desipramine, bupropion)
Probably effective
Narcolepsy
Organic mood disorders
Pseudobulbar affect (pathological laughing or crying)
Possibly effective
Personality disorders

From Rosenbaum JF, et al. *Handbook of psychiatric drug therapy.* 5th ed. Philadelphia: Lippincott Williams & Wilkins, 2005, with permission.

CHOICE OF MEDICATION

Many textbooks and articles assert that all antidepressants have roughly the same efficacy in treating depression. More recent data looking at rates of remission of depression suggest that venlafaxine and tricyclic antidepressants may be more effective than the SSRIs at achieving depression remission. The higher rates of remission are believed to be related to the combined actions of venlafaxine and TCAs on serotonin and noradrenergic systems. These effects may be achieved also by combinations of antidepressants such as bupropion and SSRIs. This complicates medication choice, as before medication choice was based mainly on symptom profile and diagnosis, prior patient response, side-effect profile, and patient tolerance. Another factor to consider when treating depression is remission rates with a particular drug. More research must be done in this area to determine the relative rates of depression remission, particularly in subtypes of patients with depression. SSRIs, bupropion, duloxetine, venlafaxine, and mirtazapine are the most well tolerated antidepressants and are generally thought of as first-line agents for major depression. Compared with TCAs and MAOIs, these medications have very low sedative, anticholinergic, and orthostatic hypotensive effects. These agents should be considered for use especially in patients with cardiac conduction disease, constipation, glaucoma, or prostatic hypertrophy.

Serotonin system

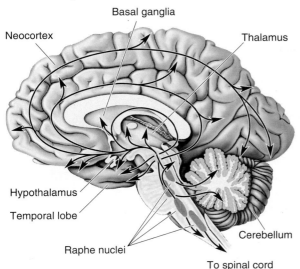

Figure 12-2 • The serotonergic diffuse modulatory systems arising from the raphe nuclei. The raphe nuclei, which are clustered along the midline of the brainstem, project extensively to all levels of the central nervous system.
From Bear MF, Connors BW, Parasido, MA. *Neuroscience—exploring the brain.* 2nd ed. Philadelphia: Lippincott Williams & Wilkins, 2001.

Among the TCAs, nortriptyline and desipramine have the least sedative, anticholinergic, and orthostatic hypotensive effects. They can be used as first-line agents in younger, healthier people, especially if cost is a consideration (tricyclics and other antidepressants available in generic form can be much less costly than newer, nongeneric medications).

Because of the necessary diet restrictions and the risk of postural hypotension, the MAOIs (phenelzine and tranylcypromine) should be used most selectively. They can be quite effective, however, and are used in patients for whom SSRIs and tricyclics have failed, in patients with a concomitant seizure disorder (MAOIs and SSRIs do not lower the seizure threshold), or in those with atypical depressions or social phobia (MAOIs or SSRIs are most effective). High-dose SSRIs and clomipramine (despite its high sedative, anticholinergic, and orthostatic hypotensive effects) are the treatments of choice for OCD.

THERAPEUTIC MONITORING

Approximately 50% of patients who meet DSM-IV criteria for major depression will recover with a single adequate trial (at least 6 weeks at a therapeutic dosage)

of an antidepressant. The most common reasons for failed trials are inadequate dose and inadequate trial length. However, dosage and length of trial are often limited by side effects (or noncompliance).

Patients on antidepressants should be monitored carefully for side effects or adverse drug reactions (listed below). Generally, antidepressant therapy of a first episode of unipolar depression should continue for 6 months. Patients with recurrent or chronic depression require longer or perhaps lifelong maintenance treatment. Increasing the dose, augmentation with lithium or T3 (Cytomel), or a psychostimulant (e.g., methylphenidate), switching antidepressants, or addition of a second antidepressant is helpful in treating refractory depression. Patients on most TCAs require serum level measurements to determine appropriate dosing.

All patients, but especially children and adolescents, should be carefully monitored for increased suicidal thinking associated with antidepressant medication treatment. While antidepressants may reduce the overall suicide rate by treating underlying depression, they may also transiently increase suicidality during periods of initiation or cessation of treatment as well as during dosage adjustments.

SIDE EFFECTS AND ADVERSE DRUG REACTIONS

SELECTIVE SEROTONIN-REUPTAKE INHIBITORS

Although specific SSRIs have slightly different side-effect profiles, as a group their main side effects are nausea, headache, neuromuscular restlessness (resembling akathisia), insomnia or sedation, and delayed ejaculation/anorgasmia. SSRIs combined with MAOIs are dangerous: a fatal serotonin syndrome may result.

TRICYCLIC ANTIDEPRESSANTS

TCAs in many patients are quite well tolerated, but because of their side effects TCAs are less well tolerated overall than are SSRIs, bupropion, or venlafaxine. The major side effects associated with TCAs are orthostatic hypotension, anticholinergic effects, cardiac toxicity, and sexual dysfunction. Specific TCAs have relative degrees of each of these effects.

Orthostatic hypotension is the most common serious side effect of the TCAs. This is particularly worrisome in elderly patients, who may be more prone to falls.

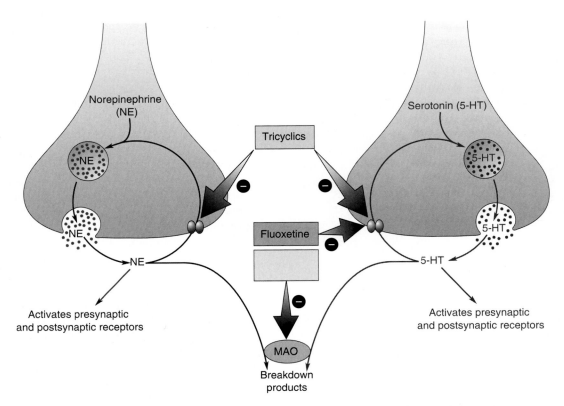

Figure 12-3 • Antidepressant drugs and the biochemical life cycles of norepinephrine and serotonin.
From Bear MF, Connors BW, Parasido, MA. *Neuroscience—exploring the brain.* 2nd ed. Philadelphia: Lippincott Williams & Wilkins, 2001.

Anticholinergic toxicity can be mild, including dry mouth, constipation, blurred near vision, and urinary hesitancy, or more severe, with agitation, motor restlessness, hallucinations, delirium, and seizures.

Cardiac toxicity may limit the use of TCAs in some patients. TCAs have quinidine-like effects on the heart, potentially causing sinus tachycardia; supraventricular tachyarrhythmias; ventricular tachycardia; ventricular fibrillation; prolongation of PR, QRS, and QT intervals; bundle branch block; first-, second-, and third-degree heart block; or ST and T-wave changes. Major complications from TCAs are rare in patients with normal hearts. TCAs should be avoided in patients with conduction system disease.

Sexual dysfunction includes impotence in men and decreased sexual arousal in women.

MONOAMINE OXIDASE INHIBITORS

Patients who take MAOIs are at risk for hyperadrenergic crises from the ingestion of sympathomimetic amines (such as tyramine) that fail to be detoxified because of inhibition of the gastrointestinal monoamine oxidase system. Improper diet can lead to severe hypertensive crises (tyramine crisis) with potential myocardial infarction or stroke. Foods that must be avoided include cured meats or fish, beer, red wine, all cheese except cottage and cream cheeses, and overripe fruits. Many over-the-counter cold and pain remedies must also be avoided. Treatment of hypertensive crisis, if severe, may require emergency medical attention, including IV phentolamine (an alpha blocker) or continuous IV nitroprusside infusion.

MAOIs cause a dose-related orthostatic hypotension: tranylcypromine can cause insomnia and agitation; phenelzine can cause daytime somnolence.

OTHER ANTIDEPRESSANTS

Venlafaxine (Effexor, Effexor XR) and duloxetine (Cymbalta) are serotonin and noradrenergic reuptake inhibitors (SNRIs) with a better side-effect profile than TCAs or MAOIs. SNRIs and TCAs may have a greater remission rate than SSRIs but further study is needed to verify superiority of broader spectrum antidepressants. Nefazodone and trazodone (Desyrel) are serotonin-modulating antidepressants. Trazodone is prescribed rarely as a sole antidepressant but is often prescribed as an adjunct to an SSRI for sleep because it has strong sedative properties (at higher doses it serves as an antidepressant). In addition to sedation, trazodone can on rare occasions induce priapism (prolonged, painful penile erection) that can cause permanent damage. Patients must be instructed to seek emergency treatment should such an erection occur. Nefazodone is similar to trazodone but is less sedating at therapeutic doses. It appears to have a low rate of sexual dysfunction but has been associated with serious hepatic abnormalities.

Bupropion (Wellbutrin, Wellbutrin SR, Zyban) appears to work by inhibiting the uptake of dopamine and norepinephrine. Bupropion has a low incidence of sexual side effects. In addition to its efficacy in treating major depression, bupropion has been shown to be effective in smoking cessation (marketed as Zyban) and attention-deficit disorder. Bupropion has a higher than average risk of seizures compared with other antidepressants. The risk of seizures is greatest above a daily dose of 450 mg or after a single dose of greater than 150 mg of immediate-release bupropion.

Mirtazapine (Remeron) is classified as a modulator of norepinephrine and serotonin. It is quite sedating in some individuals, and has a low incidence of sexual dysfunction.

PHOTOTHERAPY

Phototherapy consists of the controlled administration of bright light to treat specific psychiatric illnesses. Phototherapy is administered using specially designed bright light boxes and has been shown effective in the treatment of the seasonal subtype of major depression (also known as seasonal affective disorder) and in non-seasonal depression as well. Phototherapy is also used in the treatment of the delayed sleep phase syndrome and jet lag. In the treatment of seasonal affective disorder, early morning bright light therapy is superior to evening light in most individuals. Light intensity of 2,500 to 10,000 lux is most effective. Light therapy can induce mania in susceptible individuals.

ELECTROCONVULSIVE THERAPY

Electroconvulsive therapy (ECT), formerly known as electric shock therapy, is one of the oldest and most effective treatments for major depression. ECT also has some efficacy in refractory mania and in psychoses with prominent mood components or catatonia. ECT appears to work via the induction of generalized seizure activity in the brain. The peripheral manifestations of seizure activity are blocked by the use of paralytics, and memory for the event is blocked by the use of anesthetics and by seizure activity. Modern ECT produces short-term memory loss and confusion. Bilateral ECT is more effective than unilateral ECT but produces more cognitive side effects.

VAGUS NERVE STIMULATION

Vagus nerve stimulation (VNS) therapy is approved for treatment-refractory major depression. While the precise mechanisms of action of vagus nerve stimulation in influencing depression are unknown, it is presumed that retrograde conduction of impulses from peripheral stimulation of the nerve influence central nervous system function. Early findings suggest that VNS may influence the hippocampus, as well as the widely distributed neurotransmitters norepinephrine and gamma-amino butyric acid (GABA).

🔑 12-1 KEY POINTS

1. Antidepressants have multiple indications including various forms of depression, anxiety disorders, bulimia, and OCD, among others.
2. Antidepressants act mainly on serotonergic and noradrenergic receptor systems.
3. Some antidepressants have been shown to be efficacious for particular disorders; for major depression, all approved antidepressants reduce symptoms to a significant degree, TCAs and SNRIs may more frequently induce remission. Antidepressants for depression are often chosen based on side-effect profile and symptom constellation.
4. Some antidepressants, particularly TCAs, require monitoring of serum levels.
5. The effects of antidepressants can be augmented by the addition of lithium, thyroid hormone, or psychostimulants.
6. Antidepressants have side effects that vary according to class.
7. VNS is used for treatment-refractory depression.

References

George MS, Rush AJ, Marangell LB, et al. A one-year comparison of vagus nerve stimulation with treatment as usual for treatment-resistant depression. *Biol Psychiatry*. 2005 Sep 1;58(5):364–373.

Golden RN, Gaynes BN, Ekstrom RD, et al. The efficacy of light therapy in the treatment of mood disorders: a review and meta-analysis of the evidence. *Am J Psychiatry*. 2005 Apr;162(4):656–662.

Groves DA, Brown VJ. Vagal nerve stimulation: a review of its applications and potential mechanisms that mediate its clinical effects. *Neurosci Biobehav Rev*. 2005 May;29(3):493–500. Review.

Wagner KD. Pharmacotherapy for major depression in children and adolescents. *Prog Neuropsychopharmacol Biol Psychiatry*. 2005 Jun;29(5):819–826. Review.

Mood Stabilizers

The mood stabilizers most commonly used are lithium, valproate, carbamazepine, and lamotrigine. Table 13-1 lists mood stabilizers and their dosage and therapeutic levels. Other medications, such as calcium channel blockers and benzodiazepines, may have some utility in refractory bipolar disorder.

INDICATIONS

Mood stabilizers are indicated acutely (in conjunction with antipsychotics) for the treatment of mania. They are indicated for long-term maintenance prophylaxis against depression and mania in bipolar individuals. Anticonvulsant medications (valproate, lamotrigine, and carbamazepine) may also be useful in individuals experiencing seizure-related mood instability. Mood stabilizers are also used for treatment of impulsive behavior in individuals without bipolar disorders.

The choice of mood stabilizer is based on a patient's particular psychiatric illness (i.e., subtype of bipolar disorder) and other clinical factors such as side effects, metabolic routes, patient tolerance, and a history of patient or first-degree relative drug responsiveness. Table 13-2 lists the major mood stabilizers and their most common indications. Some common and more serious side effects of mood stabilizers are listed in Table 13-3.

The mechanism of action of mood stabilizers in bipolar illness is unclear. The range of neurotransmitters affected by these medications and their disparate modes of action suggest that mania may be controlled by altering the function of several different neurotransmitter systems. Conversely, they may share a common mechanism of action that is yet to be elucidated.

LITHIUM

MECHANISM OF ACTION

The mechanism of action of lithium in the treatment of mania is not well determined. Lithium alters at least two intracellular second messenger systems— the adenyl cyclase, cyclic adenosine monophosphate (cAMP) system, and the G protein–coupled phosphoinositide systems—and, as an ion, can directly alter ion channel function. Because norepinephrine and serotonin in the central nervous system (CNS) use G protein–coupled receptors as one of their mechanisms of action, their function is altered by lithium. Lithium also alters GABA (gamma-amino butyric acid) metabolism.

CHOICE OF MEDICATION

Lithium is indicated as a first-line treatment for regular cycling bipolar disorder in individuals with normal renal function. Lithium also is used to augment other antidepressants in unipolar depression. Lithium is renally cleared and can easily reach toxic levels in persons with altered renal function (e.g., especially elderly individuals). It is less effective in the treatment of the rapid cycling variant of bipolar disorder. When used in the treatment of mood disorders, lithium is the only intervention known to reduce suicide.

THERAPEUTIC MONITORING

Lithium levels should be monitored regularly until a stable dosing regimen has been obtained. Additional monitoring is necessary in a patient with variable

◼ TABLE 13-1 Common Mood Stabilizers[a]

Drugs	Starting Dosage	Therapeutic Dosage	Therapeutic Serum Concentration
Lithium carbonate	300 mg bid-tid	900–1500 mg/day	0.6–1.1 mEq/L
Valproic acid	250 mg bid-tid	1000–2500 mg/day	50–125 mg/L
Lamotrigine	25–50 mg qhs	300–500 mg/day	—
Carbamazepine	100 mg bid-tid	600–1200 mg/day	4–12 mg/L
Oxcarbazepine	150 mg bid	600–1200 mg/day	—
Gabapentin	300 mg qd	900–1800 mg/day	—

[a]Dosages are generally lower for geriatric patients, patients taking medications inhibiting metabolism of the drug, or patients with other medical problems.

compliance or altered renal function. In addition, patients should be warned about toxicity and be regularly assessed for side effects. Thyroid-stimulating hormone and creatinine should also be monitored at regular intervals to check thyroid and kidney function, respectively.

◼ TABLE 13-2 Psychiatric Indications for Mood Stabilizers

Drug	Uses
Lithium	Acute mania
	Long-term maintenance in bipolar disorder
	Augmentation of antidepressant medications
	Impulse dyscontrol
Valproate	Acute mania
	Rapid-cycling bipolar disorder
	Mixed features bipolar disorder
	Impulse dyscontrol
Carbamazepine	Acute mania
	Rapid-cycling bipolar disorder
	Mixed features bipolar disorder
	Impulse dyscontrol
Lamotrigine	Long-term maintenance in bipolar disorder
	Mixed features bipolar disorder

SIDE EFFECTS

Lithium has several minor but troublesome side effects, including tremor, polyuria, gastrointestinal distress, minor memory problems, acne exacerbation, and weight gain. Approximately 5% of patients on long-term lithium therapy develop hypothyroidism because the lithium interferes with thyroid hormone production. At toxic levels, ataxia, coarse tremor, confusion, coma, sinus arrest, and death can occur. Lithium has a narrow therapeutic window, and patients can become toxic at prescribed doses, especially if they undergo an abrupt change in renal function.

VALPROATE

MECHANISM OF ACTION

The mechanism of action of valproate is thought to be due in part to augmentation of GABA function in the CNS. Valproate increases GABA synthesis, decreases GABA breakdown, and enhances its postsynaptic efficacy.

CHOICE OF MEDICATION

Valproate is indicated for the treatment of acute mania and is widely used in the maintenance phase of bipolar I disorder (Table 13-2). It is more effective than lithium for the rapid-cycling and mixed variants of bipolar disorder. It may not provide prophylaxis against depression in bipolar disorder or augment antidepressants. It is used in treating impulse dyscontrol.

■ TABLE 13-3 Drugs Used as Mood Stabilizers

Drug	Side-Effect Profile	
Lithium	Therapeutic levels	
	CNS:	sedation, cognitive clouding, fine tremor
	Endocrine:	abnormal TSH, clinical hypothyroidism
	Cardiac:	T-wave change, sinus arrhythmia
	Renal:	polyuria
	Dermatologic:	acne, psoriasis
	Gastrointestinal:	nausea, vomiting, diarrhea
	Hematologic:	benign leukocytosis
	Other:	weight gain, fluid retention
	Toxic levels	
	CNS:	ataxia, coarse tremor, confusion, seizure, coma, death
	Cardiac:	sinus arrest
Valproate	Therapeutic levels	
	CNS:	somnolence, ataxia, tremor
	Endocrine:	menstrual irregularities, thyroid abnormalities
	Dermatologic:	alopecia, rash
	Hepatic:	mild transaminitis
	Gastrointestinal:	nausea, vomiting, indigestion
	Hematologic:	thrombocytopenia, platelet dysfunction
	Other:	edema
	Toxic levels	
	CNS:	ataxia, confusion, coma, death
	Cardiac:	cardiac arrest
	Idiosyncratic	
	Hepatic:	fatal hepatotoxicity
	Gastrointestinal:	pancreatitis
	Hematologic:	agranulocytosis
Carbamazepine	Therapeutic levels	
	CNS:	ataxia, sedation, dizziness, diplopia
	Dermatologic:	rash
	Cardiac:	decreased atrioventricular conduction
	Hematologic:	benign leukopenia
	Gastrointestinal:	nausea
	Toxic levels	
	CNS:	somnolence, autonomic instability, coma, death
	Cardiac:	atrioventricular block
	Respiratory:	respiratory depression
	Idiosyncratic	
	Hematologic:	agranulocytosis, pancytopenia, aplastic anemia

(Continued)

TABLE 13-3 Drugs Used as Mood Stabilizers (*continued*)

Lamotrigine	Therapeutic levels	
	CNS:	dizziness, anxiety, insomnia, somnolence, coordination abnormality, headache
	Endocrine:	dysmenorrhea
	Cardiac:	chest pain
	Dermatologic:	rash, serious life-threatening rash
	Gastrointestinal:	nausea, vomiting, dyspepsia
	Other:	weight decrease, infection, rhinitis
	Toxic levels	
	CNS:	ataxia, nystagmus, seizures, coma, death
	Cardiac:	intraventricular conduction delay

THERAPEUTIC MONITORING

Valproate levels should be monitored regularly until a stable blood level and dosing regimen have been obtained. Liver function tests should be checked at baseline and frequently during the first 6 months, especially because the idiosyncratic reaction of fatal hepatotoxicity is most frequent in this timeframe.

SIDE EFFECTS

At therapeutic levels, valproate produces a variety of side effects, including sedation, mild tremor, mild ataxia, and gastrointestinal distress. Thrombocytopenia and impaired platelet function may also occur. At toxic levels, confusion, coma, cardiac arrest, and death can occur. Valproate usage carries with it the risk of idiosyncratic but serious side effects. These include fatal hepatotoxicity, fulminant pancreatitis, and agranulocytosis.

LAMOTRIGINE

MECHANISM OF ACTION

The mechanism of action of lamotrigine in bipolar disorder is unknown. Lamotrigine is approved by the Food and Drug Administration (FDA) for use in the maintenance phase of bipolar I disorder (lamotrigine is not approved for the acute treatment of mania). Lamotrigine in vitro has been shown to inhibit voltage-sensitive sodium channels. This effect is believed to stabilize neuronal membranes and modulate presynaptic excitatory neurotransmitter release.

CHOICE OF MEDICATION

Although studies are still ongoing regarding the use of lamotrigine in bipolar disorder, it appears to be more effective in treating or preventing the depressive phase of bipolar I disorder than the manic phase.

Dosages are generally altered for elderly individuals, those with renal or other organ impairment, or when combined with interacting agents.

THERAPEUTIC MONITORING

The development of serious allergic reactions to lamotrigine appears to be related to rapid dose escalation or drug interactions. A clinically useful assay for serum levels of lamotrigine is not available. Generally, this medication should only be prescribed by a qualified psychiatrist, neurologist, or other physician who is aware of the complex drug interactions that exist particularly between valproic acid and lamotrigine.

SIDE EFFECTS

Lamotrigine can commonly cause ataxia, blurred vision, diplopia, dizziness, nausea, and vomiting. Severe, potentially life-threatening allergic rashes have been reported with the use of lamotrigine. The allergic reaction can begin as a simple rash and lead to Stevens–Johnson's syndrome. The rate of serious or life-threatening rashes is greater in the pediatric age group.

CARBAMAZEPINE

MECHANISM OF ACTION

The mechanism of action of carbamazepine in bipolar illness is unknown. Carbamazepine blocks sodium channels in neurons that have just produced an action potential, blocking the neuron from repetitive firing. In addition, carbamazepine decreases the amount of transmitter release at presynaptic terminals. Carbamazepine also appears to indirectly alter central GABA receptors.

CHOICE OF MEDICATION

Carbamazepine is generally considered to be an off-label (not FDA-approved) second-line drug (after lithium and valproate) for the treatment of mania (Table 13-2). It is used in acute mania, prophylaxis against mania in bipolar disorder, and may be more effective than lithium in rapid-cycling and mixed mania. Carbamazepine's efficacy in the prophylaxis and treatment of depression is not clear. It is also used in treating impulse dyscontrol.

SIDE EFFECTS

Carbamazepine, at therapeutic levels, produces similar CNS side effects to lithium and valproate. Nausea, rash, and mild leukopenia are also common. At toxic levels, autonomic instability, atrioventricular block, respiratory depression, and coma can occur. Carbamazepine has idiosyncratic side effects of agranulocytosis, pancytopenia, and aplastic anemia.

THERAPEUTIC MONITORING

Carbamazepine levels should be monitored regularly until a stable dosing regimen has been obtained. Patients should be carefully monitored for rash, signs of toxicity, or evidence of severe bone marrow suppression.

OXCARBAZEPINE

Oxcarbazepine is a recently-introduced anticonvulsant that is structurally similar to carbamazepine but that has fewer side effects and drug interactions. The efficacy of oxcarbazepine in treating the various stages of bipolar disorder has not been well proven. However, a few small, controlled studies suggest that oxcarbazepine is effective in acute mania. Other studies suggest the drug may be also effective in the maintenance phase of bipolar disorder.

GABAPENTIN

Gabapentin is an anticonvulsant that may be a useful adjunctive medication for anxiolysis in bipolar disorder, but it does not appear to have efficacy as a mood stabilizer as either monotherapy or when used with another mood stabilizer as adjunctive therapy. It may have efficacy as an adjunct to more traditional agents such as lithium or valproic acid or when used to address particular target symptoms such as anxiety.

ANTIPSYCHOTIC MEDICATIONS USED TO TREAT MANIA

Several atypical antipsychotic medications (Chapter 11) are also approved for use in bipolar disorder. Atypical antipsychotics approved for the mood component of bipolar disorder include olanzapine, quetiapine, risperidone, ziprasidone, and aripiprazole. Typical and atypical antipsychotics also have efficacy against the psychotic symptoms of bipolar I disorder or in psychotic unipolar depression.

🔑 13-1 KEY POINTS

1. Mood stabilizers are indicated for the treatment of bipolar disorder.
2. They work by unknown but likely varied mechanisms.
3. Efficacy varies according to the subtype of bipolar illness.
4. Mood stabilizers have serious toxicities, so patients require regular monitoring.

References

Cipriani A, Pretty H, Hawton K, et al. Lithium in the prevention of suicidal behavior and all-cause mortality in patients with mood disorders: a systematic review of randomized trials. *Am J Psychiatry.* 2005 Oct;162(10):1805–1819.

Hirschfeld RM, Kasper S. A review of the evidence for carbamazepine and oxcarbazepine in the treatment of bipolar disorder. *Int J Neuropsychopharmacol.* 2004 Dec;7(4):507–522. Review.

Yatham LN. Newer anticonvulsants in the treatment of bipolar disorder. *J Clin Psychiatry.* 2004;65 Suppl 10:28–35. Review.

Anxiolytics

The medications discussed in this chapter have anxiolysis in common. Although benzodiazepines have a wide variety of clinical applications (e.g., as preanesthetics, in the treatment of status epilepticus, as muscle relaxants, and in the treatment of insomnia) and other medications (e.g., antidepressants) are of utility in treating some forms of anxiety, the benzodiazepines are uniquely effective for the rapid relief of a broad spectrum of anxiety symptoms. Buspirone is a novel medication that, at present, is used primarily in the treatment of generalized anxiety disorder; it does not appear to be effective in treating other types of anxiety (e.g., panic).

BENZODIAZEPINES

INDICATIONS

Benzodiazepines are among the most widely used drugs in all of medicine. In psychiatry they are used as the primary treatment of a disorder or as adjunct treatment to other pharmacologic agents. Benzodiazepines are used to treat a variety of anxiety disorders: panic disorder, generalized anxiety disorder (GAD), anxiety associated with stressful life events (as in adjustment disorders with anxiety), and anxiety that complicates depression (see Chapter 3). In addition, benzodiazepines are used for the short-term treatment of insomnia, for the treatment of alcohol withdrawal, for the agitation of mania, dementia, and psychotic disorders, and in the treatment of catatonia (Table 14-1).

MECHANISM OF ACTION

Benzodiazepines appear to function as anxiolytics via their agonist action at the central nervous system (CNS) GABA$_A$ (gamma-amino butyric acid) receptors (the GABA$_A$ receptor complex regulates a chloride ion channel, GABA$_B$ receptors appear to work by second messenger systems) (Figures 14-1 and 14-2). GABA is a widespread inhibitory neurotransmitter with a complicated receptor structure, having multiple binding sites for GABA, benzodiazepines, and barbiturates. The most likely mode of action of benzodiazepines in treating psychiatric illnesses is via their augmentation of GABA function in the limbic system. Because benzodiazepines are direct agonists at a rapidly responding ion channel, their mechanism of action is virtually instantaneous with their arrival in the CNS (in contrast to buspirone, see below).

Emerging evidence in anxiety disorders suggests that altered GABA function is associated with anxiety. For example, there is evidence for reduced numbers of GABA receptors in the CNS of patients with anxiety disorders. In addition to this reduced density of GABA receptors in anxiety, the remaining GABA receptors may show decreased or altered responsiveness to benzodiazepines. There may also be reductions in the concentration of GABA in the cortex of this group. However, GABA is clearly not the only neurotransmitter implicated in susceptibility to anxiety disorders. Medications that alter monoamine function, such as serotonin and norepinephrine reuptake inhibitors, as well as buspirone (discussed below) are also highly effective in treating some anxiety disorders.

CHOICE OF MEDICATION

The selection of a benzodiazepine should be based on an understanding of potency, rate of onset, route of metabolism, effective half-life, and clinically proven effectiveness. Although all benzodiazepines appear to function by common mechanisms, the particular combination of

■ TABLE 14-1 Psychiatric Uses for Benzodiazepines

Anxiety disorders

   Generalized anxiety disorder

   Panic disorder

Mood disorders

   Temporary treatment of anxiety associated with depression

   Temporary treatment of insomnia associated with depression

   Treatment of agitation in acute mania

   Possible mood-stabilizing effect in bipolar disorder

Adjustment disorders

   Treatment of adjustment disorder with anxiety

Sleep disorders

   Short-term treatment of insomnia

Miscellaneous

   Treatment of akathisia induced by neuroleptics

   Agitation from psychosis or other causes

   Catatonia (especially lorazepam)

   Alcohol withdrawal

the above factors (and perhaps as yet unknown variations in affinity for receptor subtypes) produce varied clinical indications for different benzodiazepines. Table 14-2 illustrates the properties of some commonly used benzodiazepines and their common clinical uses.

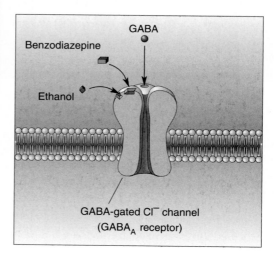

Figure 14-2 • The action of benzodiazepine. Benzodiazepines bind to a site on the GABA$_A$ receptor that makes it much more responsive to GABA, the major inhibitory neurotransmitter in the forebrain.
From Bear MF, Connors BW, Parasido, MA. *Neuroscience—exploring the brain.* 2nd ed. Philadelphia: Lippincott Williams & Wilkins, 2001.

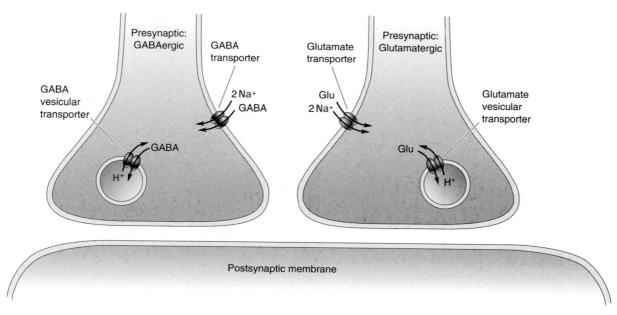

Figure 14-1 • Neurotransmitter transporters.
From Bear MF, Connors BW, Parasido, MA. *Neuroscience—exploring the brain.* 2nd ed. Philadelphia: Lippincott Williams & Wilkins, 2001.

■ TABLE 14-2 Frequently Used Benzodiazepines

Drug	Oral Dosage Equivalency (mg)[a]	Single Dosage (mg)	Usual Thera-peutic Dosage (mg/day)	Onset	Metab-olism	Elimi-nation Half-Life[b]	Active Metab	Common Uses in Psychiatry
Alprazolam (Xanax)	2	0.25–1.0	1.0–4.0	Intermed.	Oxidation	6–20	Yes	Panic, Anxiety
Chlordiaze-poxide (Librium)	40–100	5.0–25.0	15.0–100.0	Intermed.	Oxidation	30–100	Yes	Alcohol detoxi-fication
Clonazepam (Klonopin)	1	0.5–2.0	1.0–4.0	Intermed.	Oxidation	18–50	No	Panic, Anxiety
Diazepam (Valium)	20	2.0–10.0	4.0–40.0	Fast	Oxidation	30–100	Yes	Anxiety, Insomnia
Flurazepam (Dalmane)	120	15.0–30.0	15.0–30.0	Fast	Oxidation	50–160	Yes	Insomnia
Lorazepam (Ativan)	4	0.5–2.0	1.0–6.0	Intermed.	Conjugation	10–20	No	Anxiety, Catatonia
Oxazepam (Serax)	60	10.0–30.0	30.0–120.0	Slow	Conjugation	8–12	No	Alcohol Detoxi-fication
Temazepam (Restoril)	60–120	7.5–15.0	7.5–30.0	Intermed.	Conjugation	8–20	No	Insomnia
Triazolam (Halcion)	1	0.125–0.25	0.125–0.5	Fast	Oxidation	1.5–5	Yes	Insomnia

[a]Single dose equivalency.
[b]In hours. Elimination half-life includes all active metabolites.

Potency

The high-potency benzodiazepines alprazolam and clonazepam are used in the treatment of panic disorder.

Rate of Onset

Fast-onset benzodiazepines, such as diazepam, may produce a "high" feeling and are potentially more addictive. The fast-onset benzodiazepines flurazepam and triazolam are commonly used for insomnia, as is diazepam.

Route of Metabolism

All benzodiazepines listed, with the exception of lorazepam, oxazepam, and temazepam, require oxidation as a step in their metabolism. Because the oxidative functions of the liver are impaired with liver disease (e.g., cirrhosis) or with a general decline in liver function (e.g., aging), benzodiazepines that require oxidation are more likely to accumulate to toxic levels in individuals with impaired liver function.

Elimination Half-Life

The elimination half-life depicts the effective duration of action of the metabolized medications. For medications with long elimination half-lives, toxicity can easily occur with repetitive dosing. In addition, toxicology screens may remain positive for several days after the last dose of a long-acting benzodiazepine. Drugs with longer elimination half-lives offer less likelihood of inter-dose symptom rebound. For example, clonazepam is now favored over alprazolam in the treatment of panic because its longer elimination half-life provides better interdose control of panic symptoms. Medications with shorter elimination half-lives are useful for conditions such as insomnia because they are less likely to produce residual daytime sedation or grogginess.

Active Metabolites

Medications with active metabolites generally have a longer elimination half-life. Among the benzodiazepines, all but three drugs metabolized by conjugation (lorazepam, oxazepam, temazepam) and clonazepam have active metabolites.

THERAPEUTIC MONITORING

Benzodiazepine dosing is generally titrated to maximize symptom relief while minimizing side effects and the potential for abuse. No routine monitoring is required; although serum drug levels can be obtained, they are not of great clinical use. Care must be taken in prescribing benzodiazepines because of their ability to cause physiologic dependence. They cannot be discontinued abruptly due to the risk of a withdrawal syndrome that may include seizures.

SIDE EFFECTS AND ADVERSE DRUG REACTIONS

The major side effects of benzodiazepines are related to the CNS. The primary side effect of benzodiazepines is sleepiness or a general groggy feeling. Although benzodiazepines are often used to treat agitation, they may produce disinhibition (and therefore worsen agitation) in some patients (i.e., elderly individuals). Benzodiazepines are minimally depressive to the respiratory system in healthy individuals but can lead to fatal carbon dioxide retention in patients with chronic obstructive pulmonary disease. In healthy individuals, death after overdose on benzodiazepines alone is rare but does occur when benzodiazepines are taken with alcohol and other CNS depressant medications.

BUSPIRONE (BUSPAR)

INDICATIONS

Buspirone is used primarily for GAD. Because of its long lag time to therapeutic effect, patients with severe anxiety symptoms may be unable to sustain a clinical trial. Buspirone is favored as a treatment in individuals with a history of substance or benzodiazepine abuse. In general, buspirone lacks the reliability of benzodiazepines in relieving anxiety but can be effective in some people.

MECHANISM OF ACTION

Buspirone is a novel medication that appears to act as an anxiolytic via its action as an agonist at the serotonergic $5HT_{1A}$ receptor. In addition, it has some D_2 antagonist effects, although with unclear clinical significance. Unlike the benzodiazepines, it does not work rapidly; a period of several weeks of sustained dosing is required to obtain symptomatic relief. Buspirone has no GABA receptor affinity and is therefore not useful in treating benzodiazepine or alcohol withdrawal. It is not a sedative and is not useful in treating insomnia.

THERAPEUTIC MONITORING

No routine monitoring or drug levels are required when using buspirone.

SIDE EFFECTS AND ADVERSE DRUG REACTIONS

Buspirone does not tend to cause sedation, nor does it produce a significant withdrawal syndrome or dependence. The major side effects are dizziness, nervousness, and nausea.

🔑 14-1 KEY POINTS

1. Anxiolytics include benzodiazepines and buspirone.
2. Benzodiazepines bind to GABA$_A$ receptors and have a comparatively rapid onset of action; buspirone binds to serotonin receptors and takes effect after weeks of daily usage.
3. Benzodiazepines have a wide variety of uses, including anxiolysis, alcohol detoxification, agitation, and insomnia.
4. Benzodiazepines produce physiologic dependence and may manifest a significant withdrawal syndrome.
5. Buspirone treats only generalized anxiety, but does not cause physiologic dependence.

References

Gale C, Oakley-Browne M. Generalised anxiety disorder. *Clin Evid*. 2004 Dec;(12):1437–1459. Review.

O'Brien CP. Benzodiazepine use, abuse, and dependence. *J Clin Psychiatry*. 2005;66 Suppl 2:28–33. Review.

Roy-Byrne PP. The GABA-benzodiazepine receptor complex: structure, function, and role in anxiety. *J Clin Psychiatry*. 2005;66 Suppl 2:14–20. Review.

Miscellaneous Medications

This chapter includes medications that are commonly used in psychiatric practice but that do not fall into the conventional categories of psychotherapeutic drugs. Many medications used in general medical practice have side effects such as sedation, stimulation, or anxiolysis. These side effects are often exploited in psychiatry to target specific symptoms (e.g., insomnia, anergia). Other drugs, such as psychostimulants, have precise indications for psychiatric usage. Table 15-1 shows common indications of psychostimulants, anticholinergics, beta-blockers, thyroid hormones, and other drugs. Many more medications than are discussed here are included in the psychiatric armamentarium.

PSYCHOSTIMULANTS

Psychostimulants are used in psychiatry to treat attention-deficit disorder, narcolepsy, and some forms of depression. Commonly used psychostimulants are dextroamphetamine (Dexedrine), methylphenidate (Ritalin), Adderall (a mixture of amphetamines), and pemoline (Cylert). The mechanism of action of these medications appears to occur through their alterations of central nervous system (CNS) monoamine function. Their primary mechanism of action is thought to be facilitating endogenous neurotransmitter release (rather than acting as a direct agonist). Psychostimulants have the liabilities of inducing tolerance and psychological dependence, which may lead to abuse. The side effects of these medications are due largely to their sympathomimetic actions and include tachycardia, insomnia, anxiety, hypertension, and diaphoresis. Weight loss may be an unwanted side effect in young children but a desirable one in overweight adults.

ATOMOXETINE

Atomoxetine (Strattera) is a selective norepinephrine reuptake inhibitor medicine approved for treating attention-deficit disorder. Similar medications are approved in other countries for treating depression and atomoxetine is used off-label in the United States for treating depression. However, the efficacy of atomoxetine in depression is unknown. Like other medications that have monoamine reuptake as a primary mechanism of action (e.g., selective serotonin-reuptake inhibitors, SSRIs), atomoxetine has been associated with an increased risk of suicide in children and adolescents and requires careful monitoring, especially during the initiation or tapering of therapy.

ANTICHOLINERGICS

Medications with anticholinergic activity are commonly used in psychiatry to treat or provide prophylaxis for some types of neuroleptic-induced movement disorders. Anticholinergics are generally used as first-line agents in the treatment of neuroleptic-induced parkinsonism and for acute dystonia; they may also have some utility in treating akathisia but are best tried after beta-blockers and lorazepam. The most commonly used anticholinergics are benztropine and trihexyphenidyl. In addition, diphenhydramine, an antihistamine that also possesses anticholinergic properties, is frequently used to treat neuroleptic-induced movement disorders and to provide nonspecific sedation. These medications are CNS muscarinic antagonists. Side effects of anticholinergics, due to peripheral anticholinergic action, include blurry vision (as a result of cycloplegia), constipation, and urinary retention; their principal central

TABLE 15-1	Psychiatric Uses of Miscellaneous Medications
Medication	**Major Psychiatric Uses**
Psychostimulants	Treatment of attention-deficit disorder
	Treatment of depression in elderly or medically ill individuals
	Treatment of narcolepsy
	Augmentation of antidepressants in refractory depression
Anticholinergics	Treatment of neuroleptic-induced parkinsonism
	Treatment of neuroleptic-induced dystonia
Beta-blockers	Treatment of impulsivity
	Treatment of performance anxiety
	Treatment of akathisia
	Treatment of lithium-induced tremor
Disulfiram	Prevention of alcohol ingestion
Opioid Antagonist	Treatment of alcoholism
Glutamate Modulator	Treatment of alcoholism
Opioid Partial Agonist	Treatment of opiate dependence
Clonidine	Treatment of impulsivity
	Treatment of Tourette's syndrome
	Treatment of opiate withdrawal
	Treatment of attention-deficit disorder
Acetylcholinesterase Inhibitors	Treatment of mild to moderate memory loss in Alzheimer's disease
NMDA Antagonist	Treatment of moderate to severe memory loss in Alzheimer's disease
Thyroid Hormones	Augmentation of antidepressants in refractory depression

side effects are sedation and delirium. Anticholinergic toxicity is a major cause of delirium, especially in individuals with dementia and human immunodeficiency virus (HIV) encephalopathy.

BETA-BLOCKERS

Beta-blockers are used widely in general medicine. In psychiatry, they have a few specific uses. Beta-blockers likely alter behavior and mood states by altering both central and peripheral catecholamine function. For example, in anxiety, they may diminish central arousal; peripherally, they may reduce tachycardia, tremor, sweating, and hyperventilation. Common side effects of beta-blockers include bradycardia, hypotension, asthma exacerbation, and masked hypoglycemia in diabetics. Beta-blockers may also produce depression-like syndromes characterized by fatigue and depressed mood.

NALTREXONE

Naltrexone (ReVia) is a *mu* opioid antagonist that is used to prevent alcohol relapse and to lessen the severity of a relapse in individuals with alcohol dependence. Naltrexone treatment is initiated once a patient has been detoxified from alcohol. For individuals co-abusing opiates or who are receiving opiates for medical reasons, naltrexone treatment should not be initiated until at least 1 week after the last opiate exposure (an opiate antagonist can precipitate severe opiate withdrawal if given to opiate-dependent persons). Naltrexone reduces alcohol craving, reduces the probability of an alcohol relapse, and reduces the severity of a relapse when one occurs. Naltrexone, like all treatments for alcohol dependence, works best when combined with psychosocial interventions.

ACAMPROSATE

Acamprosate (Campral) is the most recently approved medication used in the treatment of alcohol dependence. Acamprosate is indicated for maintaining abstinence in previously alcohol-dependent subjects who are abstinent at treatment initiation. Acamprosate may work via numerous mechanisms, including as a modulator of glutamate function. This medication seems to reduce the craving and urge to drink in patients recently withdrawn from alcohol and helps maintain abstinence and make relapse less severe. Acamprosate should be combined with psychosocial interventions in the treatment of alcoholism.

DISULFIRAM (ANTABUSE)

Disulfiram is used to prevent alcohol ingestion through the fear of the consequences of ingesting alcohol while taking disulfiram (Table 15-1). Disulfiram blocks the oxidation of acetaldehyde, a step in the metabolism of alcohol. The buildup of acetaldehyde produces a toxic reaction, making an individual who ingests alcohol while taking disulfiram severely ill within 5 to 10 minutes. Symptoms include flushing, headache, sweating, dry mouth, nausea, vomiting, and dizziness. In more severe reactions, chest pain, dyspnea, hypotension, and confusion occur. Fatal reactions, although rare, can occur. Disulfiram use should be restricted to carefully selected patients who are highly motivated and who fully understand the consequences of drinking alcohol while taking disulfiram. Side effects in the absence of alcohol ingestion include hepatitis, optic neuritis, and impotence.

BUPRENORPHINE

Buprenorphine is used for the treatment of opiate addiction. As a partial opioid agonist, buprenorphine has a role in opiate detoxification. Unlike methadone maintenance treatment for opiate dependence (which can only be used in specialized methadone treatment centers), oral buprenorphine (Subutex), or a formulation containing buprenorphine and naloxone (Suboxone) are available for use in outpatient office-based practices. The parental form of buprenorphine (Buprenex) is used intramuscularly for treating symptoms of opiate withdrawal in some circumstances. Because buprenorphine is a partial opioid agonist, it has a greater safety margin with regard to side effects such as respiratory depression. Mixing buprenorphine with naloxone is designed to prevent diversion of the buprenorphine tablets for recreational intravenous injection. If taken as an oral sublingual preparation as prescribed, the naloxone (an opiate antagonist) in the medication has poor absorption and therefore does not interfere with the desired therapeutic effect of buprenorphine. However, if the oral pill is crushed or otherwise converted to an injectable form, the naloxone component (as a mu opioid antagonist) is effective, blocking naloxone's effects as a partial agonist at the mu opioid receptor.

CLONIDINE

Clonidine is a CNS alpha$_2$ adrenoreceptor agonist. The alpha$_2$ adrenoreceptor is a presynaptic autoreceptor that inhibits the release of CNS norepinephrine. The primary use of clonidine in medicine is as an antihypertensive (Table 15-1). In psychiatry, clonidine has been variously used. It is effective in decreasing autonomic

symptoms associated with opiate withdrawal, in the treatment of attention-deficit disorder (ADD) and Tourette's syndrome, and may be useful for impulsiveness and other forms of behavioral dyscontrol. Side effects include sedation, dizziness, and hypotension.

COGNITIVE ENHANCERS

Donepezil (Aricept), rivastigmine (Exelon), galantamine (Reminyl), and tacrine (Cognex) are reversible inhibitors of the enzyme acetylcholinesterase and are used to enhance cognition in patients with mild to moderate dementia of the Alzheimer's type. Rivastigmine also inhibits butyrylcholinesterase, a property that may contribute greater efficacy to rivastigmine in later stages of Alzheimer's disease. Galantamine also has activity at nicotinic cholinergic receptors that may be clinically significant. Some of the cognitive deficits in Alzheimer's disease are due to loss of cholinergic neurons in the basal forebrain that project to the cerebral cortex and hippocampus, which results in a deficiency of cholinergic neurotransmission (Figure 15-1). By inhibiting the enzyme or enzymes that hydrolyze synaptic acetylcholine, these drugs are thought to raise synaptic concentrations of acetylcholine in the remaining cholinergic neurons. Initially, these drugs reduce cognitive

Acetylcholine system

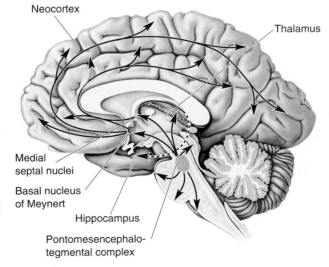

Figure 15-1 • The cholinergic diffuse modulatory systems arising from the basal forebrain and brainstem.
From Bear MF, Connors BW, Parasido, MA. *Neuroscience—exploring the brain.* 2nd ed. Philadelphia: Lippincott Williams & Wilkins, 2001.

impairment; however, this effect wanes with the progressive loss of cholinergic neurons. Common side effects include gastrointestinal upset and other cholinomimetic effects including bradycardia and increased gastric acid secretion. Tacrine can cause elevations in serum transaminases and severe hepatotoxicity, and is therefore reserved for second-line treatment.

MEMANTINE (NAMENDA)

Memantine is an antagonist at the excitatory glutamatergic N-methyl-D-aspartate (NMDA) receptor. Memantine is approved for the treatment of moderate-to-severe dementia of the Alzheimer type. Antagonism of the NMDA receptor may help prevent glutamate-mediated excitotoxicity and improve function of neurons involved in some forms of memory (e.g., the hippocampus).

THYROID HORMONES

Thyroid hormones are used primarily in psychiatry to augment the effects of antidepressants. They also may be used as adjuncts in treating rapid cycling bipolar disorder.

Although clinical hypothyroidism can mimic the symptoms of depression, some individuals without clinical hypothyroidism may respond to thyroid augmentation. The theoretic basis for using thyroid hormones lies in the finding of altered hypothalamic–pituitary–adrenal axis functioning in depressed individuals. Although there is debate as to their relative efficacy, both T_3 (tri-iodo thyronine) and T_4 (tetra-iodo thyronine) cross the blood–brain barrier. T_4 has been shown to be of use in conjunction with lithium to improve clinical control of rapid cycling bipolar disorder. Side effects at low doses are minimal; when dosages result in over-replacement, symptoms of hyperthyroidism emerge.

15-1 KEY POINTS

1. Miscellaneous medications are widely used for treatment of symptoms and side effects.
2. They overlap with medications used in other medical practice.
3. The medications have side effects and efficacy specific to each medication and its target symptoms.

References

Boothby LA, Doering PL. Acamprosate for the treatment of alcohol dependence. *Clin Ther.* 2005 Jun;27(6):695–714.

Doody RS. Refining treatment guidelines in Alzheimer's disease. *Geriatrics.* 2005 Jun;Suppl:14–20. Review.

Fudala PJ, Woody GW. Recent advances in the treatment of opiate addiction. *Curr Psychiatry Rep.* 2004 Oct;6(5):339–346. Review.

Kaduszkiewicz H, Zimmermann T, Beck-Bornholdt HP, et al. Cholinesterase inhibitors for patients with Alzheimer's disease: systematic review of randomised clinical trials. *Br Med J.* 2005 Aug 6;331(7512):321–327. Review.

Major Adverse Drug Reactions

This chapter describes a group of major adverse reactions associated with use of psychiatric medications. Minor adverse reactions and side effects are outlined in the chapters on the respective medications. Although the adverse drug reactions discussed below (with the exception of serotonin syndrome) are most commonly produced by antipsychotic medications, they may occur in response to other medications. The major adverse drug reactions to antipsychotics, their risk factors, onset, and treatment are outlined in Table 16-1. Although the *Diagnostic and Statistical Manual of Mental Disorders*, 4th edition, classifies dystonia, akathisia, extrapyramidal symptoms (EPS), neuroleptic malignant syndrome (NMS), and tardive dyskinesia as neuroleptic-induced movement disorders, it is clear that akathisia can occur with the use of non-neuroleptic psychiatric medications.

DYSTONIA

Dystonia is a neuroleptic-induced movement disorder characterized by muscle spasms. Dystonia commonly involves the musculature of the head and neck but may also include the extremities and trunk. Symptoms may range from a mild subjective sensation of increased muscle tension to a life-threatening syndrome of severe muscle tetany and laryngeal dystonia (laryngospasm) with airway compromise. The muscle spasms may lead to abnormal posturing of the head and neck with jaw muscle spasm. Spasm of the tongue leads to macroglossia and dysarthria; pharyngeal dystonia may produce impaired swallowing and drooling. Ocular muscle dystonia may produce oculogyric crisis.

Risk factors include use of high-potency antipsychotics, with young men at increased risk. The condition usually develops early in drug therapy (within days).

Treatment of dystonia depends on the severity of the symptoms. In the absence of laryngospasm or severe patient discomfort, intramuscular (IM) anticholinergic medication (benztropine or diphenhydramine) can be used. In more severe cases or if laryngospasm is present, intravenous (IV) anticholinergic medication is used. Some cases may require intubation if respiratory distress is severe. Discontinuation of the precipitating antipsychotic is sometimes necessary; in other cases, the addition of anticholinergic medications on a standing basis prevents the recurrence of dystonia.

AKATHISIA

Akathisia, a common side effect produced by antipsychotic medications, is also caused by serotonin-reuptake inhibitors. Akathisia consists of a subjective sensation of inner restlessness or a strong desire to move one's body. Individuals with akathisia may appear anxious or agitated. They may pace or move about, unable to sit still. Akathisia can produce severe dysphoria and anxiety in patients and may drive them to become assaultive or to attempt suicide. It is important to diagnose akathisia accurately because if mistaken for agitation or worsening psychosis, antipsychotic dosage may be increased with resultant worsening of the akathisia.

Risk factors for akathisia include a recent increase in medication dosing or the recent onset of medication use. Most cases occur within the first month of drug therapy but can occur at any time during treatment.

Treatment consists of reducing the medication (if possible) or using either beta-blockers (propanolol is commonly used) or benzodiazepines (especially lorazepam). Although there is some debate regarding their efficacy, anticholinergics (diphenhydramine or benztropine) are also used frequently.

■ TABLE 16-1 Neuroleptic-Induced Movement Disorders[a]

Disorder	Risk Factors	Onset	Treatment
Dystonia	High-potency antipsychotics Young men	First few days of therapy	IM/IV benztropine or diphenhydramine Severe laryngospasm may require intubation
Akathisia	Recent increase/onset of medication dosing	First month of therapy	Propanolol, lorazepam (maybe anticholinergics)
EPS	High-potency antipsychotics Elderly Prior episode of EPS	First few weeks of therapy	Anticholinergics Lowering antipsychotic dosage or changing to lower-potency antipsychotic
NMS	High-dose antipsychotics, rapid dose escalation, or IM injection of antipsychotics Agitation, dehydration Prior episode of NMS	Usually within first few weeks; can occur at any point in antipsychotic therapy	Discontinuing antipsychotic medication Supportive symptom management Dantrolene, bromocriptine May require intensive care
TD	Elderly Long-term antipsychotic treatment Female African American Mood disorders	Usually after years of treatment	Lowering dosage of antipsychotic Changing antipsychotics Changing to Clozaril

[a]The DSM-IV classification for these disorders defines them as neuroleptic-induced movement disorders. The term *neuroleptic* generally refers to typical antipsychotics (see Chapter 11). Exceptions include risperidone, which is classified as an atypical antipsychotic but can cause all the above disorders; selective serotonin-reuptake inhibitors, which are not neuroleptic drugs but can clearly produce akathisia; and Clozaril, which does not appear to produce dystonia, akathisia, EPS, or TD but may cause NMS.

EXTRAPYRAMIDAL SYMPTOMS

EPS, also known as neuroleptic-induced parkinsonism, consist of the development of the classic symptoms of Parkinson's disease but in response to neuroleptic use. The most common symptoms are rigidity and akinesia, which occur in as many as half of all patients receiving long-term neuroleptic therapy. A 3- to 6-Hz tremor may be present in the head and face muscles or the limbs. Akinesia or bradykinesia are manifested by decreased spontaneous movement and may be accompanied by drooling. Rigidity consists of the classic parkinsonian "lead pipe" rigidity (rigidity that is present continuously throughout the passive range of motion of an extremity) or cogwheel rigidity (rigidity with a catch and release character).

Risk factors for the development of EPS include the use of high-potency neuroleptics, increasing age, and a prior episode of EPS. EPS usually develops within the first few weeks of therapy.

Treatment consists of reducing the dosage of antipsychotic (if possible) and adding anticholinergic medications to the regimen.

NEUROLEPTIC MALIGNANT SYNDROME

NMS is an idiosyncratic and potentially life-threatening complication most commonly associated with antipsychotic drug use. However, NMS may occur spontaneously, in response to any medication that blocks dopamine receptors, and in response to reductions or changes in dopamine agonist medications. Symptoms of NMS may develop gradually over a period of hours to days and can often overlap with symptoms of general

■ **TABLE 16-2** Neuroleptic Malignant Syndrome

Autonomic
  Tachycardia, other cardiac arrhythmias
  Hypertension
  Hypotension
  Diaphoresis
  Fever progressing to hyperthermia
Motor
  Rigidity/dystonia
  Akinesia
  Mutism
  Dysphagia
Behavioral
  Agitation
  Incontinence
  Delirium
  Seizures
  Coma
Laboratory
  Increased creatine kinase
  Abnormal liver function tests
  Increased white blood cell count

medical illness. The major clinical findings in patients with NMS are presented in Table 16-2. Many symptoms of NMS are nonspecific and overlap with symptoms common to other psychiatric and medical conditions. The diagnosis of NMS is also complicated by the waxing and waning nature of the clinical picture.

Autonomic instability coupled with motor abnormalities is essential to the diagnosis of NMS. Autonomic alterations can include cardiovascular alterations with cardiac arrhythmias and labile blood pressure. Low-grade fever progressing to severe hyperthermia may also be present. Motor findings may overlap with other motor abnormalities in psychiatric illness; for example, rigidity/dystonia can be confused with simple dystonia or with EPS. Mutism can be a sign of severe psychosis or catatonia alone, although this does occur with NMS. Behavioral features such as agitation can also overlap with other psychiatric syndromes; however, the presence of delirium or seizures is a harbinger of more serious general medical illness (including drug withdrawal) or NMS. Laboratory findings may reveal an increased creatine kinase secondary to myonecrosis from sustained muscular rigidity. Liver enzymes may be elevated, but their relation to NMS is unclear. Leukocytosis is also often present.

Risk factors for the development of NMS (Table 16-1) include the use of high-dose antipsychotics, rapid dose escalation, intramuscular (IM) injection of antipsychotics, dehydration, agitation, or a prior history of NMS. Some factors may be related to severity of illness (e.g., severely ill patients often have poor oral intake and become dehydrated, are more likely to be placed in restraints, and require IM injection of an antipsychotic) rather than causative factors. Although NMS is most common during the first few weeks of antipsychotic drug therapy, it can occur at any time during therapy.

Treatment of this potentially fatal disorder is largely supportive. Specific interventions include discontinuation of antipsychotics (an option that may take a long period of time in individuals treated with depot antipsychotics); restoration of recently withdrawn dopamine agonists; dantrolene (a muscle relaxant) is used to treat rigidity and decrease myonecrosis; and bromocriptine (a dopamine agonist) is sometimes used to reverse dopamine-blocking effects of antipsychotics or other anti-dopaminergic medications. Symptom management including intensive care with cardiac monitoring and intubation may be necessary. Symptoms of NMS overlap with serotonin syndrome (Table 16-3). However, in NMS, muscular rigidity and increased creatine kinase are prominent. In addition, serotonin syndrome develops in response to the use of medications that affect serotonin function (especially monoamine oxidase inhibitors, MAOIs), whereas NMS develops in response to anti-dopaminergic medications. In patients using both MAOIs and antipsychotics (e.g., refractory psychotic depression), the differential diagnosis can be quite difficult.

TARDIVE DYSKINESIA

Tardive dyskinesia (TD) is a movement disorder that develops with long-term neuroleptic use; rarely, especially in elderly individuals, onset may not be as delayed. TD consists of constant, involuntary, stereotyped choreoathetoid movements most frequently confined to the head and neck musculature. At times, the extremities and respiratory and oropharyngeal musculature are also involved.

Risk factors include long-term treatment with neuroleptics, increasing age, female sex, and the presence of a mood disorder. Although TD is reversible in some cases, it tends to be permanent.

TABLE 16-3 Serotonin's Syndrome

Autonomic
  Tachycardia
  Hypertension
  Diaphoresis
  Fever progressing to hyperthermia
Motor
  Shivering
  Myoclonus
  Tremor
  Hyperreflexia
  Oculomotor abnormalities
Behavioral
  Restlessness
  Agitation
  Delirium
  Coma

Treatment consists of changing antipsychotics, lowering the dosage, or switching to clozapine. Clozapine, which appears to work by a mechanism different from other antipsychotics, may reduce or eliminate the abnormal movements of TD.

SEROTONIN'S SYNDROME

Serotonin's syndrome results from high synaptic concentrations of serotonin. The syndrome can result from a single use of medications or illicit drugs that alter serotonergic function but most commonly occurs when multiple medications that alter serotonin metabolism are used. Classically, this syndrome is produced when other serotonin-altering medications are used with MAOIs. This syndrome, which can be life-threatening, consists of symptoms outlined in Table 16-3. These include severe autonomic instability, motor abnormalities,

and behavioral changes. The course of the disorder can exist on a continuum from very mild symptoms to becoming malignant and ending in coma and death. A similar syndrome occurs when MAOIs are used with meperidine or dextromethorphan, and perhaps other opiates.

Serotonin's syndrome has many similarities to NMS, but clues to the differential diagnosis may arise from the history of medication exposure and the clinical symptoms. NMS occurs following or during the use of antipsychotic medication; while serotonin syndrome occurs through use of MAOIs or other serotonergic agents. NMS tends to have a gradual onset while serotonin syndrome can be abrupt. Serotonin's syndrome may present with shivering, hyperreflexia, and clonus. Prominent gastrointestinal symptoms (e.g., nausea and diarrhea) may suggest serotonin syndrome. Muscular rigidity can develop in severe cases of serotonin syndrome, thus mimicking NMS.

Risk factors for serotonin syndrome, other than combining MAOIs with other serotonin-altering medications, are not known.

Treatment for serotonin syndrome is largely supportive and may require intensive care with cardiac monitoring and mechanical ventilation. The serotonin 2A receptor antagonist cyproheptadine shows efficacy in treating this condition. The offending medications should be discontinued.

🔑 16-1 KEY POINTS

1. Major adverse drug reactions occur most commonly in psychiatry with use of antipsychotics and serotonin-altering medications.
2. Antipsychotics can cause dystonia, akathisia, EPS, NMS, and TD.
3. Serotonin-altering medications can cause akathisia and serotonin syndrome.
4. All of the above adverse drug reactions are reversible, except for TD, which may be permanent.

References

Bhanushali MJ, Tuite PJ. The evaluation and management of patients with neuroleptic malignant syndrome. *Neurol Clin*. 2004 May;22(2):389–411. Review.

Boyer EW, Shannon M. The serotonin syndrome. *N Engl J Med*. 2005 Mar 17;352(11):1112–1120. Review.

Sachdev PS. Neuroleptic-induced movement disorders: An overview. *Psychiatr Clin North Am*. 2005 Mar;28(1): 255–274. Review.

17 Psychological Theories

There are a large number of competing theories influencing contemporary psychotherapeutic thinking. Psychotherapies derived from psychoanalytic, cognitive, and behavioral theories are the most widely used. Cognitive-behavioral interventions and interpersonal therapy have the strongest empirical verification; little empirical evidence supports the efficacy of analytic/dynamic therapies.

PSYCHOANALYTIC/ PSYCHODYNAMIC THEORY

The principal theorist responsible for launching psychoanalysis as a technique and psychodynamic theory in general is Sigmund Freud. Freud's theories proposed that unconscious motivations and early developmental influences were essential to understanding behavior. Freud's original theories have proved quite controversial and have led to the creation of various alternative or derivative theories.

TWENTIETH-CENTURY SCHOOLS OF PSYCHODYNAMIC PSYCHOLOGY

There are three major twentieth-century psychodynamic schools: drive psychology, ego psychology, and object relations theory.

Drive Psychology

Drive psychology posits that infants have sexual (and other) drives. This theory proposes that sexual and aggressive instincts are present in each individual and that each individual passes sequentially through psychosexual developmental stages (oral, anal, phallic, latency, and genital). Included in drive psychology is conflict theory, which proposes to explain how character and personality development are influenced by the interaction of drives with the conscience and reality.

Ego Psychology

Freud eventually developed a tripartite theory of the mind in which the psychic structure was composed of the id, ego, and superego. Under this theory, the id is the compartment of the mind containing the drives and instincts. The superego contains the sense of right and wrong, largely derived from parental and societal morality. The ego is responsible for adaptation to the environment and for the resolution of conflict. A major function of the ego is the reduction of anxiety. Ego defenses (Table 17-1) are proposed as psychic mechanisms that protect the ego from anxiety. Some ego defenses (e.g., sublimation) are more functional for the individual than others (e.g., denial).

Object Relations Theory

Object relations theory (*objects* refers to important people in one's life) departs from drive theory in that the relationship to an object is motivated by the primacy of the relationship rather than the object being a means of satisfying a drive. Child observation furthered object relations theory, emphasizing concepts of attachment and separation.

The interpersonal school arose as an outgrowth of object relations theory. The interpersonal theorists emphasize that intrapsychic conflicts are less important than one's relationship to one's sense of self and to others. In other words, the relationships in a person's

■ TABLE 17-1 Common Ego Defense Mechanisms

Denial	Feelings or ideas that are distressing to the ego are blocked by refusing to recognize evidence for their existence.
Projection	Feelings or ideas that are distressing to the ego are attributed to others.
Regression	Feelings or ideas that are distressing to the ego are reduced by behavioral return to an earlier development phase.
Repression	Feelings or ideas that are distressing to the ego are relegated to the unconscious.
Reaction formation	Feelings or ideas that are distressing to the ego are converted into their opposites.
Displacement	Feelings or ideas that are distressing to the ego are redirected to a substitute that evokes a less intense emotional response.
Rationalization	Feelings or ideas that are distressing to the ego are dealt with by creating an acceptable alternative explanation.
Suppression	Feelings or ideas that are distressing to the ego are not dealt with, but they remain components of conscious awareness.
Sublimation	Feelings or ideas that are distressing to the ego are converted to those that are more acceptable.

Modified from Sadock BJ, Sadock VA. *Comprehensive textbook of psychiatry.* 7th ed. Philadelphia: Lippincott Williams & Wilkins, 1999.

life are given primary importance in producing happiness or misery. Interpersonal psychotherapy (IPT) for depression and related conditions has good empirical validation and may work as well as medication treatment and possibly better than cognitive-behavioral therapy (CBT).

ERIKSON'S LIFE CYCLE THEORY

Erik Erikson made major contributions to the concept of ego development. Erikson theorized that ego development persists throughout one's life, and conceptualized that psychosocial events drive change, leading to a developmental crisis. According to Erikson's model, individuals pass through a series of life cycle stages (Table 17-2). Each stage presents core conflicts produced by the interaction of developmental possibility with the external world. Individual progress and associated ego development occur with successful resolution of the developmental crisis inherent in each stage. This model allows for continued ego development until death.

COGNITIVE THEORY

Cognitive theory recognizes the importance of the subjective experience of oneself, others, and the world. It posits that irrational beliefs and thoughts about oneself, the world, and one's future can lead to psychopathology.

In cognitive theory, thoughts or cognitions regarding an experience determine the emotions that are evoked by the experience. For example, the perception of danger in a situation naturally leads to anxiety. When danger is truly present, anxiety can be adaptive, leading to hypervigilance and self-protection. When the situation is only perceived as dangerous (such as in fear of public speaking), the resulting anxiety can be psychologically paralyzing. A person may fear public speaking because of an irrational fear that something disastrous will occur in public. A principal type of irrational belief is a cognitive distortion (Table 17-3).

BEHAVIORAL THEORY

Behavioral theory posits that behaviors are fashioned through various forms of learning, including modeling, classical conditioning, and operant conditioning (Table 17-4). A behaviorist might propose that, through operant conditioning, depression is caused by a lack of positive reinforcement (as may occur after the death of a spouse), resulting in a general lack of interest in behaviors that were once pleasurable (or reinforced).

COGNITIVE-BEHAVIORAL THERAPY

Cognitive and behavioral theories form part of the bases of CBT. CBT involves the examination of cognitive distortions and the use of behavioral techniques to treat common disorders such as major depression. CBT has strong empirical validation and is effective in

■ TABLE 17-2 Erikson's Life Cycle Stages

Trust vs. mistrust	Birth to 18 mo	The infant has many needs but does not have the power to have those needs met. The child is dependent on caretakers. If care taking is appropriate, a sense of trust and hope are created. If inappropriate or inadequate, mistrust develops.
Autonomy vs. shame	18 mo to 3 y	The child is learning about the use of language and control of bowel and bladder function and walking. As a result, it begins to choose to influence and explore the world. If care taking is appropriate, the child will develop a healthy balance between exerting its autonomy and feeling shame over the consequences of exerting autonomy.
Initiative vs. guilt	3–5 y	As the child develops increasing control of language and walking, he or she has increased initiative to explore the world. The potential for action carries with it the risk of guilt at indulging forbidden wishes.
Industry vs. inferiority	5–13 y	The child begins to develop a sense of self based on the things he or she creates. Caretaker influences are important in helping the child develop a sense of mastery and competence over creating.
Identity vs. role confusion	13–21 y	Corresponds to adolescence. How one appears to others is important in this stage. There are conflicts between one's identity and the need to gain acceptance.
Intimacy vs. isolation	21–40 y	The anxiety and vulnerability produced by intimacy are balanced against the loneliness produced by isolation.
Generativity vs. stagnation	40–60 y	If successful, the individual develops a positive view of his or her role in life and a sense of commitment to society at large. If unsuccessful, individuals move through life without concern for the greater welfare.
Ego integrity vs. despair	60 y to death	An individual accepts his or her life course as appropriate and necessary. If this fails, the individual may regret or wish to relive some part of life, leading to despair.

Modified from Sadock BJ, Sadock VA. *Comprehensive textbook of psychiatry.* 7th ed. Philadelphia: Lippincott Williams & Wilkins, 1999.

■ TABLE 17-3 Types of Cognitive Distortions

Arbitrary inference	Drawing a specific conclusion without sufficient evidence
Dichotomous thinking	A tendency to categorize experience as "all or none"
Overgeneralization	Forming and applying a general conclusion based on an isolated event
Magnification/ minimization	Over- or undervaluing the significance of a particular event

Modified from Sadock BJ, Sadock VA. *Comprehensive textbook of psychiatry.* 7th ed. Philadelphia: Lippincott Williams & Wilkins, 1999.

■ TABLE 17-4 Important Concepts in Behavior Theory

Modeling	A form of learning based on observing others and imitating their actions and responses
Classical conditioning	A form of learning in which a neutral stimulus is repetitively paired with a natural stimulus, with the result that the previously neutral stimulus alone becomes capable of eliciting the same response as the natural stimulus
Operant conditioning	A form of learning in which environmental events (contingencies) influence the acquisition of new behaviors or the extinction of existing behaviors

the treatment of depression, social phobia, obsessive–compulsive disorder, posttraumatic stress disorder (PTSD), and panic disorder. CBT and pharmacotherapy, such as antidepressant medications, are generally thought to be synergistic, particularly with regard to the treatment of depression. However, CBT as a treatment appears to have long-lasting effects in terms of preventing relapse that have not been well demonstrated with medication treatment for most conditions.

DIALECTICAL-BEHAVIORAL THERAPY

Dialectical behavioral therapy (DBT) is a psychotherapy developed specifically for the treatment of borderline personality disorder in females. The foundation of DBT resides in CBT principles, but the therapy encompasses empirical findings from multiple areas of psychology, sociology, Zen philosophy, and dialectical philosophy. Overall, DBT focuses on therapist and patient acceptance of the patient as the foundation for developing skills for behavioral and emotional change. DBT has

strong empirical support in the treatment of borderline personality disorder and is the first-line psychotherapy for treating this condition.

🔑 17-1 KEY POINTS

1. Psychological theories are numerous, but those derived from psychoanalytic, cognitive, and behavioral theories are most widely used.
2. The psychoanalytic school emphasizes unconscious motivations and early influences.
3. The object relations school emphasizes the importance of relationships with other people.
4. The cognitive school emphasizes subjective experience, beliefs, and thoughts.
5. The behavioral school emphasizes the influence of learning.
6. CBT and IPT have the greatest empirical support for treating depression and anxiety.

References

de Mello MF, de Jesus Mari J, Bacaltchuk J et al. A systematic review of research findings on the efficacy of interpersonal therapy for depressive disorders. *Eur Arch Psychiatry Clin Neurosci.* 2005 Apr;255(2):75–82.

Hollon SD, Stewart MO, Strunk D. Enduring effects for cognitive behavior therapy in the treatment of depression and anxiety. *Annu Rev Psychol.* 2006;57: 285–315.

Robins CJ, Chapman AL. Dialectical behavior therapy: current status, recent developments, and future directions. *J Personal Disord.* 2004 Feb;18(1):73–89.

18 Legal Issues

Legal issues affect all areas of medicine, including psychiatry. The laws that govern medical practice address physician duty, negligence, and malpractice as well as patient competence or capacity, consent, and right to refuse treatment. Previous court decisions, or precedents, are used as the standard by which a given action (or inaction) is judged. Practitioners should be aware of the pertinent laws of the state in which they practice in order to comply adequately with standards of practice while respecting the rights and duties of their role. Reducing adverse events and legal claims in the health care system is known as risk management.

MALPRACTICE

The legal definition of malpractice requires the presence of four elements: negligence, duty, direct causation, and damages. Negligence can be thought of as failure to perform some task with respect to the patient, falling short of the care that would be provided by the average practitioner (the standard of care). Duty reflects the law's recognition of the obligation of the physician to provide proper care to his or her patients. Direct causation requires that the negligence directly caused the alleged damages. Finally, damages (e.g., physical or emotional harm) must in fact be shown to have occurred. In short, malpractice involves the negligence of a duty that directly causes damages. Malpractice claims in psychiatry principally involve suicides of patients in treatment, misdiagnosis, medication complications, false imprisonment (involuntary hospitalization or seclusion), and sexual relations with patients.

INFORMED CONSENT

Informed consent has three elements: information, capacity, and consent. First, appropriate levels of information regarding a proposed treatment, including side effects, alternative treatments, and outcome without treatment, must be provided (the process of informing or disclosing). Second, the patient must have capacity, i.e., possess the ability to understand, appreciate, reason, and express a choice (make decisions) regarding the risks and benefits of treatment. Third, the patient must give consent voluntarily (important to the concept of volition is the lack of subtle or overt coercion). The elements of informed consent and capacity are depicted in Figure 18-1. True emergency situations are an exception to this rule; treatments necessary to stabilize a patient in an emergency can be given without informed consent. (Commonly, the word *capacity* is used to describe a patient or research volunteer's ability to make a treatment or research participation decision. *Competence*, generally, refers to the findings of a judicial or other legal proceeding regarding a person's ability to consent. However, the two terms are often used interchangeably.) It is important to realize that individuals who have psychiatric disorders such as major depression, mild dementia, or schizophrenia may still retain capacity to consent to treatment or research interventions. All that is required is that a person meet the aforementioned criteria for capacity.

INVOLUNTARY COMMITMENT

Commitments are generally judicially supported actions that require persons to be hospitalized or treated against their will. Although laws vary from

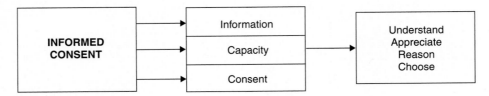

Figure 18-1 • The elements of informed consent and capacity.

state to state, commitment criteria usually require evidence that the patient is a danger to self, a danger to others, or is unable to care for himself or herself. Psychiatrists, in most localities, have the right to commit a patient, temporarily and involuntarily, if any of these criteria are met and a diagnosis of a mental disorder is provided (in other words, both a mental disorder and danger must exist). The duration of temporary commitment and the rights of the patient vary by jurisdiction. Patients who have been committed have a right to be treated, and unless they have been declared incompetent, they have the right to refuse treatment.

THE TARASOFF DECISIONS: DUTY TO WARN (OR PROTECT)

Tarasoff v The Board of Regents of the University of California (or simply, *Tarasoff*) was a landmark case that was heard twice in the California Supreme Court in 1976. Tarasoff I held that therapists have a duty to warn the potential victims of their patients. Tarasoff II held that therapists have a duty to take reasonable steps to protect potential victims of their patients. In most localities, this means that the therapist should take reasonable action to protect a third party if a patient has specifically identified the third party and a risk of serious harm seems imminent. However, there are many different legal interpretations of the duty to warn. Such varying interpretations of the responsibilities of physicians regarding the balance between confidentiality and protecting others create great difficulty in psychiatric practice. Because the specific legal requirements vary by state law, it is important to understand the requirements of each jurisdiction.

M'NAGHTEN RULE: THE INSANITY DEFENSE

Named after a mentally ill man (M'Naghten) who attempted to assassinate the prime minister of England in 1843, this rule forms the basis of the insanity defense. According to the M'Naghten rule, a person is not held responsible for a criminal act if at the time of the act he or she suffered from mental illness or mental retardation *and* did not understand the nature of the act *or* realize that it was wrong. In more recent history, the appropriate use of the insanity defense has been called into question. Some legal theorists argue for the designation "guilty but insane" to indicate culpability but at the same time recognize the presence of a mental illness (and presumably the need for treatment).

18-1 KEY POINTS

1. Malpractice consists of negligence, duty, direct causation, and damages.
2. The essential elements of informed consent are information, capacity, and consent.
3. The *Tarasoff* decision led to an expectation that therapists and doctors take reasonable action to protect persons whom their patients have specifically threatened.
4. The M'Naghten rule is the basis of the insanity defense.

References

Kachigian C, Felthous AR. Court responses to Tarasoff statutes. *J Am Acad Psychiatry Law.* 2004;32(3):263–273. Review.

Kim SY. Evidence-based ethics for neurology and psychiatry research. *NeuroRx.* 2004 Jul;1(3): 372–377. Review.

Moye J, Gurrera RJ, Karel MJ et al. Empirical advances in the assessment of the capacity to consent to medical treatment: Clinical implications and research needs. *Clin Psychol Rev.* 2005 Aug 30; [Epub ahead of print].

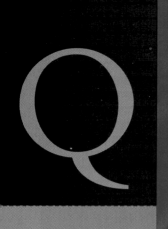

Questions

1. A physician is very attentive and compassionate with his patients. One of his patients sustains a permanent injury that would not have occurred if the physician had made the correct diagnosis. The physician finished his residency more than 20 years ago and the diagnosis has only been well-established for the past 5 years. On questioning, the physician is unaware of the diagnosis. You are asked to review the case. Which of the following elements is evidenced by this physician's unfamiliarity with the diagnosis?
   a. Duty
   b. Direct causation
   c. Damages
   d. Failure to meet standard of care
   e. Poor risk management

2. a 20-year-old man with schizophrenia has recently had a change in his antipsychotic medication. His delusions and hallucinations are now well controlled, but he is complaining of some muscular rigidity. Which of the following agents would be an appropriate choice of address this new problem?
   a. Methylphenidate
   b. Benztropine
   c. Pemoline
   d. Atenolol
   e. Clonidine

3. A 26-year-old woman presents with a multiple complaints. She has recently completed a workup for a seizure disorder. No abnormalities were detected on neurologic evaluation. She has been followed in a pain clinic for management of pain in her neck, lower back, knees, and head. She has been evaluated by an orthopaedic surgeon but no underlying etiology could be identified. She reports that she has been unable to attain orgasm for several years. She further reports a long history of difficulty swallowing and numerous dietary restrictions. This presentation is most consistent with which of the following?

   a. Somatization disorder
   b. Conversion disorder
   c. Pain disorder
   d. Hypochondriasis
   e. Body dysmorphic disorder

4. A 5-year-old white boy is brought to your office because of problems sleeping. The parents report that they have witnessed the child sit up in bed with a frightened expression and scream loudly. He appears awake and intensely frightened, but then falls back asleep and has no memory of the event. This disturbance most likely occurs during what phase of sleep?
   a. Stage 0
   b. Stage 2
   c. Delta
   d. REM
   e. Stage 1

5. A 45-year-old white woman presents with a 1-year history of the following symptoms: sweating, trembling, sensation of choking, chest discomfort, lightheadedness, derealization, fear of losing control, and fear of dying. The symptoms develop over about 10 minutes in situations where the patient feels trapped. The patient has been largely disabled by the symptoms. She has been unable to pick up her children at school, go shopping, or engage in her normal social events. She would like to avoid using any type of medication. You begin by teaching relaxation exercises and desensitization combined with education aimed at helping the patient understand that her panic attacks are the result of misinterpreting bodily sensations. What is the name of this technique?
   a. Exposure therapy
   b. Psychodynamic therapy
   c. Biofeedback therapy
   d. Cognitive-behavioral therapy
   e. Classical conditioning

6. The patient described above becomes impatient with the progress of her psychotherapy. She now requests psychopharmacologic management. She has been reading about the disorder and has some familiarity with its pharmacologic management. Of the appropriate medications, you choose a medication that acts as an agonist at the GABA receptor. Which of the following medications meet these criteria?
   a. Alprazolam
   b. Mirtazapine
   c. Imipramine
   d. Paroxetine
   e. Phenelzine

7. A 22-year-old white woman with a prior diagnosis of bulimia nervosa presents to the emergency room during her college exam period with an irregular heartbeat. The patient is weighed and found to be at her ideal weight. She has been treated with sertraline and states that she has been taking it as prescribed. On examination the patient is noted to have a callus on the second joint of the right index finger. The electrocardiogram demonstrates a flattening of the T waves with development of U waves. What is the most likely finding?
   a. Hypokalemia
   b. Hyperkalemia
   c. Hypercalcemia
   d. Hypocalcemia
   e. Esophageal rupture

8. Some of the cognitive deficits in Alzheimer's disease are due to loss of cholinergic neurons in the basal forebrain that project to the cerebral cortex and hippocampus. One of the current mainstays of therapy is to increase the effectiveness of acetylcholine transmission in the remaining neurons. What is the mechanism by which donepezil and tacrine achieve this?
   a. Binding to the acetylcholine postsynaptic receptor
   b. Irreversibly binding acetylcholinesterase
   c. Presynaptically blocking reuptake of acetylcholine
   d. Reversibly inhibiting acetylcholinesterase
   e. Acting as a postsynaptic agonist

9. A 48-year-old woman who lives in a state-supported group home presents to the Emergency Department after having a witnessed grand mal seizure shortly after dinner. She is lethargic and disoriented upon arrival and gradually becomes more alert during your assessment. She tells you that she does not remember what happened. A staff member from the group home tells you that the patient has been under stress lately and has been drinking a large amount of diet cola. Her medicines include clozapine 500 mg qhs, lithium 500 mg tid, glycopyrrolate (Robinul)

2 mg qhs, and escitalopram 20 mg qd. Her blood pressure is elevated at 195/95. Her heart rate is 90 and her respiratory rate is 15. She does not smoke. A basic electrolyte laboratory panel reveals a serum sodium of 119. Her chest x-ray is normal. What is the most likely diagnosis?
   a. Syndrome of inappropriate antidiuretic hormone secretion (SIADH)
   b. Clozapine toxicity
   c. Hypertensive encephalopathy
   d. Primary polydipsia
   e. Serotonin's syndrome

10. A 24-year-old woman presents for a routine physical examination. You are running late and have kept her waiting for 40 minutes alone in the examination room. She is staring down at the floor when you arrive. Apologizing, you begin to review her medical history. She begins to cry and then suddenly gets angry when you ask whether the nurse took her vitals. She says "I was having such a nice conversation with her and then she just left and never returned." You explain that there are many other patients in your primary care office today and that she had to go and see other patients. Sensing that she is still having difficulties, you ask her what is going on in her life. She tells you that her boyfriend of 2 months left her abruptly last month and she has not been able to stop crying. You query her about neurovegetative symptoms (such as depressed mood, decreased interests or pleasure, appetite change or weight loss or gain, sleep disturbance, psychomotor agitation or retardation, fatigue or low energy, worthlessness or guilt, impaired concentration or decision making, thoughts of death or suicide), and she endorses some symptoms but not enough to diagnose major depression. She clearly brightens in response to your attention to her feelings and you begin examining her. She has numerous scratch marks on her upper thighs, some of which appear old and some more recent. You ask how she got them and her eyes avert to the floor again. "I did them," she states. "It makes the pain bearable." You finish her examination and refer her to a colleague for a psychiatric consultation. From your recollections from your own psychiatric training in medical school, you suspect she will be diagnosed with:
    a. Narcissistic personality disorder
    b. Major depression
    c. Borderline personality disorder
    d. Generalized anxiety disorder
    e. Sexual masochism

11. A 45-year-old divorced man is referred to you from his company's employee assistance program because he is on probation at his job. You are asked to evaluate him for the presence of a mental illness that could be affecting his performance. He arrives for the appointment 15 minutes

late and looks annoyed with you. You explain to him that his evaluation is confidential but that if there is information that he would like shared with his employer to help provide accommodations, you could provide such information. He goes on to explain that he has been fired from or left several jobs in the past because his co-workers failed to recognize his unique talents. In each situation he describes feeling as if he could have led the organization better and that, in fact, he should be the boss. He is surprised when you ask what qualities he has that he thinks sets him apart. He blushes a bit, appearing humiliated and then snaps back it you, "what do you know about business leadership, you're a doctor?" You explain that you were curious about the nature of his talents. He noticeably calms and then confesses that he really does not have any talents and begins to cry. You listen and talk some more and then complete your evaluation. He denies neurovegetative signs of depression and exhibits no manic signs or symptoms. What is the most likely diagnosis?

a. Schizoid personality disorder
b. Delusional disorder, grandiose subtype
c. Borderline personality disorder
d. Narcissistic personality disorder
e. Dependent personality disorder

12. You are asked by the nurse at your clinic to conduct a home visit on a reclusive 47-year-old woman who has been unable to come in for an appointment for the last 3 years. Her daughter agrees to meet you at the home the next morning. She shows you into the house where you find the patient sitting in a house dress in a reclining chair in her living room. She tells you that she has not left the house in 3 years "because it is too scary out there," gesturing toward the street. You ask more about what happened 3 years ago. She recounts that she was out at a shopping center when she suddenly had the abrupt onset of a severe wave on anxiety. It lasted approximately 15 minutes but caused her to run out of the mall and back to the safety of her car. Since then, she has had many more such attacks. She has refused to leave her home for the last 2$\frac{1}{2}$ years. She says that she likes having people visit her but she just can't bring herself to go out again. She has the attacks sometimes at home and has not sought treatment for them. She said that the same thing happened to her mother and she spent the rest of her life at home. She asks you if you understand what is going on with her and can you fix it? You tell her that you have seen this before and can recommend the right kinds of treatment. The primary condition is:

a. Major depression
b. Panic disorder
c. Generalized anxiety disorder
d. Arachnophobia
e. Obsessive–compulsive disorder

13. A 9-year-old boy is brought into the emergency department (ED) by his distraught parents after trying to attack his mother with a kitchen knife. His mother was unharmed but the parents called the police who suggested an emergency evaluation after observing their son's demeanor. He was verbally aggressive and pacing, talking loudly, and swearing. The police escorted them to the ED. The boy was restrained and medicated acutely in the ED with a combination of emergency sedatives. The parents explain to you that their son seemed to develop attention-deficit disorder a few months ago and was prescribed a dextro-amphetamine-containing medication by his pediatrician. It seemed to help at first, but then his personality began to change. Where before he was an affable, bright, athletic boy, he became increasingly wary, agitated, and sleepless. The situation worsened recently when he started accusing his mother of putting poison in his food. He attacked his mother after she made a new dish with which he was unfamiliar. The patient's father has bipolar disorder. His maternal uncle has schizophrenia and his mother had attention-deficit/hyperactivity disorder as a child. The best next step would be to hospitalize the patient and:

a. Start citalopram therapy
b. Start lithium therapy
c. Start aripiprazole therapy
d. Start group therapy
e. Discontinue dextro-amphetamine therapy

14. An 8-year-old girl presents for a pediatric visit because her teacher has raised concerns about her lack of talking at school. Her mother tells you that her daughter talks all the time at home and has many interests and activities. She also describes her daughter as having achieved all developmental milestones at appropriate ages. However, when she is at school she does not speak spontaneously and will only speak when spoken to directly by her teacher. She is having difficulty socially as she does not reciprocate social interactions with her peers. When she is at home she plays actively with her two sisters and talks normally. What do you tell the mother her daughter suffers from?

a. Major depression
b. Posttraumatic stress disorder
c. Autism
d. Selective mutism
e. Abulia

15. A 27-year-old nurse appears in a private physician's office complaining of recurrent back pain. On exam, the patient is noted to have a runny nose, dilated pupils, piloerection, mild fever, and mild tachycardia. The patient reports that she has previously used oxycodone for her back pain for brief periods but has not used any pain relievers for several months. She states that she has back problems "about twice a year." You obtain an additional laboratory test,

make a diagnosis, and prescribe treatment for this patient. A week later, you are the emergency ward attending physician when the patient is brought in by ambulance unconscious with very slow respirations and mild perioral cyanosis. The best emergency treatment for this patient is:

a. Flumazenil
b. Physostigmine
c. Clonidine
d. Acamprosate
e. Naloxone
f. Alprazolam
g. Thiamine
h. Glucose

16. A 4-year-old boy whose family recently emigrated from another country is brought in by his parents for an initial visit with the pediatrician. The child had not started school in his country and his parents have been alarmed by his failure to reach developmental milestones. He has developed physically but has been slow in his development of language skills and has extreme difficulty following instructions. You find him in good physical shape and note that he makes good eye contact with you but appears confused by what you are trying to do. He also cries and reaches for his mother several times when you are trying to examine him. You refer him for neuropsychological testing and the results reveal an Intelligence Quotient of 62. Upon your next visit, you tell the parents his diagnosis and prognosis. They are:

a. Severe mental retardation, will need institutional care
b. Mild mental retardation, is educable but will need extra support
c. Autistic disorder, will need special education
d. Asperger's syndrome, will be able to function with support
e. Moderate mental retardation

17. An 88-year-old woman is brought into the emergency room by her daughter because of a change in her mental status. She had been previously doing well until she was left at home with her daughter's husband for a week while the daughter was away on business. You examine her and order a head computerized tomogram (CT). The head CT reveals a subdural hematoma that appears to be less than a week old. There also is soft-tissue swelling over her cranium and around her jaw. You suspect elder abuse and order an x-ray series looking for other fractures. The x-ray series reveals several recent fractures of the ribs and long bones of her body. After consulting a neurosurgeon about the need for subdural drainage, the next best step is to:

a. Call the risk management officer for the hospital
b. Call social services for a consult
c. Call the son-in-law at home and confront him

d. Call the local police to have the daughter arrested
e. Refer her back to her primary care physician and send her home

18. A 39-year-old woman walks into the emergency department with a broken nose. She tells you that she fell out of bed and landed on her face. She and her husband both smell of alcohol but do not appear intoxicated. You obtain a surgical consult, and after the patient is evaluated, you check in with her again. Before you enter the room, you overhear the husband speaking in a threatening tone to his wife. He says "you deserved it this time you louse!" When you enter the room, he appears startled and she appears frightened. You suspect spousal abuse. The best next step would be to:

a. Call the police to arrest the husband
b. Pull the husband out of the room and confront him
c. Try to separate the couple and talk to the woman alone
d. Call the patient's home to see if anyone there knows what happened
e. Ask the couple more about how she fell out of the bed

19. A 28-year-old man from the local state hospital is brought into the emergency department mute and in a rigid posture. He has a core temperature of 101°F, a blood pressure of 200/110, heart rate of 128, and is able to move all four extremities distally and proximally, and responds to deep tissue pain, but little else. You obtain an old discharge summary from a surgical admission from 2 years ago for appendicitis. In it you find mention that the patient was taking olanzapine, haloperidol, fluoxetine, trazadone, and valproic acid. You order a complete metabolic serum panel. His creatine phosphokinase (CPK) comes back severely elevated at 110,000 units per liter. His blood pressure becomes unstable and you move him to the intensive care unit. The most likely diagnosis is:

a. Serotonin's syndrome
b. Neuroleptic malignant syndrome
c. Dystonia
d. Tardive dyskinesia
e. Pneumonia

20. A 22-year-old man presents to your office pacing and speaking rapidly. Your nurse tries to get him to calm down and wait for you but is unable. She asks you to see him immediately. When you enter the room, he jumps up and starts rambling about going to medical school and being especially gifted. He describes no longer needing sleep, mastering speed reading, and spending money on expensive clothes for his new career. He asked you what he should wear when he wins the Nobel prize for medicine. After gathering more history from his family, you decide that he is acutely manic. The medication most likely to help his condition is:

a. Flumazenil
b. Fluoxetine
c. Acamprosate
d. Gabapentin
e. Valproic acid

21. A 3-year-old boy is evaluated in the pediatric general practice clinic because his mother thinks he's "too quiet." She notes specifically that her pregnancy and delivery were uncomplicated. A few months after birth she noted that her child did not seem to respond to her attempts to communicate with him. He failed to respond when smiled at, had almost no facial expressions, and didn't maintain eye contact. He didn't babble or begin talking like other children his age, but used only occasional odd-sounding phrases in a repetitive fashion. In addition, she worries that he sits for hours rocking back and forth. He doesn't play with other children, and overall shows little interest in his external world. The most likely diagnosis is:
a. Autistic disorder
b. Childhood-onset schizophrenia
c. Conduct disorder
d. Attention-deficit disorder
e. Separation-anxiety disorder

22. A 48-year-old woman is interviewed in the emergency department after her sister brought her in because she was afraid her sister might "do something crazy." The sister reports that the patient has been depressed for a very long time, and that she has been undergoing serious stress. She states that the patient has been saying she would be better off dead, and that life isn't worth living. The patient reports that she has been progressively more depressed during the past month. She recounts stressors of losing her job 1 month ago due to cutbacks, but she believes they let her go because she wasn't performing well. In addition, 3 weeks ago she ended a long-term romantic relationship of 5 years after a great deal of anger and turmoil. A week prior to admission she learned that her previously rent-controlled apartment where she had lived for many years was being sold and that she would have to move. She loves her neighborhood, but won't be able to afford living there any longer. She reports that she has felt seriously depressed for at least 1 month, and has had marked neurovegetative symptoms of depression. In addition, she reports a profound sense of anhedonia, and spends her days lying in bed without eating or showering. She notes that she is hopeless about the future, and that she doesn't believe she will ever feel better. She is vague when directly questioned about suicidality. You make the diagnosis of major depression, but you are concerned about the patient's suicide risk. The most important risk factor for suicide in this patient is:
a. Major depression
b. Neurovegetative symptoms

c. Loss of a romantic relationship
d. Loss of her job
e. Hopelessness

23. A 24-year-old man with a history of schizoaffective disorder presents in your primary care office with his mother for a routine physical exam. He tells you that he was recently hospitalized for the fourth time in the last year for paranoia. His psychiatrist started him on a new medication, but then the patient forgot his first follow-up appointment. His physical examination is normal. You counsel him on smoking cessation and order a routine complete blood count. Then, 2 days later, you notice that his white blood count came back at a low 1.9. You ask that the patient be brought into your office for re-evaluation and page his psychiatrist. The most likely antipsychotic agent the patient has been taking is:
a. Risperidone
b. Aripiprazole
c. Clozapine
d. Quetiapine
e. Thioridazine

24. A 39-year-old man visits a new primary care physician for a first visit at the urging of his mother. He denies symptoms of depression except for occasional low mood. His father died when he was 14 and he has lived with his mother since that time. He works as a computer programmer and says that he has many acquaintances but few friends and no romantic relationships. His mother had to convince him to go to the appointment because he had trouble deciding to see a physician. His mother accompanies him on the visit and relays that she often decides things for him because he has "never been able to think for himself." He says, "People think I'm too clingy. The truth is I just want people to care about me." When you speak with him alone, he appears to have a normal intellect, no magical or odd thinking, and a stable sense of self but reveals a desperate fear that his mother will abandon him. He denies any self-destructive or impulsive behaviors. The most likely diagnosis is:
a. Borderline personality disorder
b. Dependent personality disorder
c. Schizotypal personality disorder
d. Narcissistic personality disorder
e. Personality disorder

25. A 27-year-old woman is brought to the emergency department by the local police because she has been harassing her neighbors. Her family arrives shortly afterward and appears very concerned. The police report that the young woman's apartment manager called because she was banging on all her neighbors' doors and screaming in the stairwell. Upon examining the patient's apartment, the

police found the place to be filthy and malodorous, with rotting garbage and food in the kitchen. The windows were sealed and covered with dark curtains, and there were several televisions and computers in the living room, all turned on at the same time. The patient's family reports that for the past year or so she has seemed increasingly odd, disassociated herself from family activities, and gave up a well-paying job as a computer system administrator. In addition, she had abruptly ended a long-term romantic relationship for no particular reason. On mental status examination the young woman is disheveled and wearing several layers of dirty clothes. She appears wary and guarded. Her speech is normal in rate, volume, and production. She is conversant, and explains that she has been defending herself against aliens who want to use her as a specimen. She believes that she began picking up on hidden transmissions in her e-mail at work, revealing an alien conspiracy, perhaps involving the CIA. She states that she left her job to monitor these hidden transmissions full-time and that she has been hiding in her apartment because they know she is on to them. She ended her recent relationships because she felt that the aliens would harm the people she cared about. She denies substance use or any medical symptoms. She reports that she has been eating and sleeping well, and that her mood is good. She denies hearing voices. Diagnostic testing, including drug screen, complete blood count, chemistry panel, and brain MRI are all normal. The most likely diagnosis is:

a. Schizophrenia
b. Bipolar disorder
c. Major depression
d. Alcohol abuse
e. Paranoid personality disorder

26. A 35-year-old man is seen in a prison clinic for a routine physical exam. He tells you that he is in jail for murdering two people in a botched robbery attempt. When you ask him about his other criminal history, he relays numerous arrests and some convictions for theft, assault, drunk driving, and rape. Penal records indicate a persistent pattern of lying and theft while incarcerated and that he exhibits no remorse when caught by authorities. He has never been psychiatrically hospitalized and denies any episodes of elevated, expansive, or fluctuating mood. He exhibits no grandiosity, pressured speech, or psychotic symptoms. Family history is significant for alcohol dependence in his father and mother and for no history of bipolar disorder. He calmly reports that his father and subsequent foster parents often beat him with straps or boards when he was a child. He was knocked unconscious on several occasions but has no history of seizures and denies nightmares or flashbacks from the abuse. He has had suicidal ideation but has not made suicide attempts or been self-destructive. The most likely diagnosis is:

a. Conduct disorder
b. Posttraumatic stress disorder
c. Cyclothymic disorder
d. Bipolar disorder
e. Antisocial personality disorder

27. A 19-year-old man is seen on rounds on a psychiatric unit after being admitted two nights before. He was diagnosed with psychotic disorder, not otherwise specified and begun on risperidone 1 mg twice per day. The nurse asked you to see him first because he had been "agitated all morning." When you enter his room, you find him pacing the floor. He tells you that he feels restless and that he has to keep moving to feel better. Other than pacing, he is not exhibiting any tremors or other movements of the extremities. Although he appears agitated, his psychotic symptoms, which include hallucinations and delusions, do not appear to have worsened since admission. Vital signs are within normal limits and he is afebrile. A serum CPK is drawn and is normal. The most likely diagnosis is:

a. Dystonia
b. Parkinsonism
c. Akathisia
d. Neuroleptic malignant syndrome
e. Tardive dyskinesia

28. A 15-year-old boy is brought to his pediatrician's office because his parents are embarrassed by his behavior. They report that he has been intermittently barking and yelping repetitively during conversations. This behavior persists in public and at school. In addition, he has periods of bizarre body posturing with jerky upper extremity movements and snorts like a horse. His parents believe he is punishing them for setting limits on television and social time with his friends. The young man denies any retaliation against his parents. He states that he develops a powerful urge to bark and yelp, and that other times he finds himself moving uncontrollably. He is upset about his behaviors and feels like a "freak." The most likely reason for the young man's behavior is:

a. Adolescent rebellion
b. Schizophrenia
c. Substance abuse
d. Tourette's disorder
e. Conduct disorder

29. A 41-year-old man with a 21-year history of bipolar disorder comes to the emergency department with ataxia, coarse tremor of his upper extremities, confusion, and diarrhea. He reports that he has been sweating a great deal because it is "so hot outside" and that he "gets no relief" at home because his halfway house is not air-conditioned. His medications are fluoxetine 40 mg per day, lithium carbonate 300 mg each morning and 600 mg

each evening, oxcarbazepine 300 mg each morning and 900 mg each evening, olanzapine 7.5 mg each evening, and lorazepam 1 mg per day. He denies having used any illicit drugs. On examination, his heart rate is 100 and regular, blood pressure is 98/60, respiratory rate is 14, and temperature is 98.7°F. The most likely diagnosis is:

a. Lithium toxicity
b. Lorazepam toxicity
c. Fluoxetine toxicity
d. Oxcarbazepine toxicity
e. Serotonin's syndrome

30. An 18-year-old college student is brought to the emergency room by the campus police due to creating a disturbance on campus. On examination he has auditory hallucinations, agitation, and rapid, incoherent speech. The length of time that he has had the symptoms is unknown. Substance abuse history is unknown. The most likely diagnosis is:

a. Schizophreniform disorder
b. Winter depression
c. Generalized anxiety disorder
d. Atypical depression
e. Obsessive–compulsive disorder

31. A 23-year-old man is psychiatrically evaluated in the surgical intensive care unit after sustaining a self-inflicted gunshot wound to the abdomen. The patient is conscious but sedated following surgical intervention. On examination, the patient is vague and guarded. He provides a history that he was not suicidal and that he accidentally shot himself while cleaning the gun. He admits to drinking a few beers before the incident. At this point, the next step in properly evaluating this patient is:

a. To accept the patient's assertion that the event was accidental
b. To obtain a head CT
c. To obtain a thyroid stimulating hormone level
d. To refer the patient to Alcoholics Anonymous
e. To obtain additional history from the patient and family, friends, or witnesses to the event

32. Additional history obtained from a close friend reveals that the patient in the previous question had been despondent over a romantic breakup and worsening performance in college. The patient did not ingest alcohol routinely, but had drunk to the point of intoxication at least twice in the past week. The patient's family reported that he had been avoiding them over the past few days. Based on the additional history, it seems reasonable to:

a. Accept the patient's assertions that the gunshot was accidental
b. Discuss your findings with the patient and explain that you are concerned about the possibility of a suicide attempt

c. Discuss the patient's alcohol abuse with the patient
d. Keep your findings secret from the patient so as not to provoke anger at his friends and family
e. Initiate pharmacological treatment with an antidepressant medication

33. You prescribe a selective serotonin-reuptake inhibitor antidepressant for a patient suffering from major depression requiring an inpatient psychiatric admission; 2 days later the patient appears markedly anxious. The nursing staff is very concerned, suggesting the patient may need additional sedation. On your exam the patient is agitated and pacing, bouncing her legs up and down during your interview and is unable to focus on the conversation. She notes that she doesn't know what is happening, but that she just can't sit still, feeling like she has to move her legs around. The most likely diagnosis is:

a. Neuroleptic malignant syndrome
b. Medication-induced akathisia
c. Generalized anxiety disorder
d. Serotonin's syndrome
e. Caffeine intoxication

34. A 53-year-old man admitted to the inpatient psychiatric unit for treatment of bipolar disorder is found lying in the hallway. On exam, he is conscious, but is confused and dysarthric. The staff reports that he has been progressively sedated and confused for the past 24 hours. He states: "I think the doctors are trying to kill me." Upon reviewing his chart, you note that he was admitted 1 week prior and restarted on his usual dose of carbamazepine due to a low level. Then, 3 days ago, he developed an upper respiratory infection and was treated with an antibiotic. His last carbamazepine level was 3 days ago. You conduct a thorough physical and review of systems to assure yourself that the patient did not suffer a syncopal episode and wasn't injured when he fell. The most likely diagnosis is:

a. Malingering
b. Dementia
c. Drug toxicity
d. Progressive upper respiratory infection
e. Normal pressure hydrocephalus

35. A 22-year-old man who recently was fired from his job as an auto mechanic presents in the emergency room complaining of a conspiracy against him at his former workplace. When he first begins to explain the situation it sounds like possible workplace harassment. You think about referring him to a lawyer when he informs you that his boss is an alien emperor from Jupiter and that his co-workers are the emperor's loyal subjects. When you ask him to describe the situation more, he coherently elaborates a richly detailed story about the aliens at the garage and how they conspired to eliminate him. Other than

these unusual beliefs, he appears normal in terms of dress and body posture. The most likely subtype of schizophrenia in this patient is:

a. Paranoid
b. Catatonic
c. Disorganized
d. Undifferentiated
e. Residual

36. You are asked to see a 27-year-old man who was discharged 2 days ago from a psychiatric hospital. The nurse reports to you that the patient has developed a hand tremor that looks like he is rolling a pill. He also tells you that the patient is walking very stiffly and appears to be having trouble initiating his movements. Which of the following medications would be most likely to have caused the condition above?

a. Lorazepam
b. Benztropine
c. Quetiapine
d. Clozapine
e. Haloperidol

37. A 43-year-old male is admitted to the hospital for a leg fracture sustained after falling from a ladder while intoxicated with alcohol. He reports a history of daily alcohol use since the age of 9 years except for rare periods of sobriety during brief stints in jail or in hospitals. He is currently taking opiate pain relievers for leg pain and is receiving thiamine, folate, and benzodiazepines for alcohol withdrawal. Appropriate management at this point would include:

a. Continue his current treatment regimen with downward adjustments in opiate and benzodiazepine dosing as pain and alcohol withdrawal symptoms subside
b. Add naltrexone to his current treatment regimen to treat alcohol dependence
c. Stop opiate pain relievers because he may become addicted to them
d. Stop benzodiazepines because he may become addicted to them
e. Add an antidepressant medication to his current treatment regimen

38. The patient recovers nicely from his fracture and has a successful detoxification from alcohol. He has not required opiate pain relievers or benzodiazepines for the past week. The patient expresses an interest in future treatment options for alcohol dependence. The best treatment recommendation would include:

a. Alcoholics Anonymous (AA), cognitive-behavioral therapy (CBT), and naltrexone
b. Naltrexone monotherapy
c. CBT

d. AA
e. Duloxetine monotherapy
f. Oxazepam monotherapy
g. Acamprosate monotherapy

39. A 20-year-old woman who presented to your office 1 month ago with postpartum depression returns for follow-up. She states that her mood improved shortly after beginning fluoxetine. Her energy is greatly improved. She states she has cleaned her house several times and is only sleeping 2 to 3 hours each night. She is speaking quickly and appears distractible. The most appropriate treatment would be:

a. Increase her fluoxetine
b. Schedule electroconvulsive therapy
c. Begin a mood stabilizer and stop fluoxetine
d. Begin dialectical behavioral therapy
e. Begin cognitive-behavioral therapy

40. A 50-year-old mentally retarded patient with schizophrenia presents to the emergency room with airway obstruction. On presentation the patient is hypoxic. Emergency personnel ascertain that the patient has an upper airway obstruction and will require an emergency tracheotomy. What would be the critical issues regarding informed consent with this patient?

a. Providing an appropriate level of information for a patient with mental retardation and schizophrenia
b. Establishing competence in a hypoxic mentally retarded patient with schizophrenia
c. Ensuring that the consent is voluntary
d. The patient should be committed
e. Informed consent is not necessary

41. A 45-year-old black man presents 3 months after a myocardial infarction he sustained at his place of employment where he works as the head chef. For the past month he has been having trouble concentrating and remembering his recipes. He complains of decreased interest and pleasure in his work and hobbies. He has also has difficulty falling asleep at night. He has had very little energy despite successful cardiac rehabilitation. He has lost 20 lbs during this time. The symptoms are threatening his job and his relationship with his wife. The most appropriate agent for initial treatment of this condition would be:

a. Electroconvulsive therapy
b. Tricyclic antidepressant
c. Lithium
d. Monoamine oxidase inhibitor
e. Selective serotonin-reuptake inhibitor

42. A 30-year-old woman presents with the chief complaint that everyone always leaves her. She has been married and divorced three times. She states that each husband

initially seemed perfect, but she subsequently realized they were total fakes. She reports that her parents divorced when she was 4 and that she was raped by her stepfather numerous times from the ages of 6 to 10. She has had over 60 sexual partners. She reports persistent financial concerns. She expresses chronic feelings of emptiness. During the interview, the patient is alternately seductive and irritable. She has a history of a polysubstance abuse, but denies any recent substance abuse history. The most appropriate treatment for this patient is:

a. Begin antipsychotic medication
b. Electroconvulsive therapy
c. Dialectical behavioral therapy
d. Inpatient psychiatric admission to a dual diagnosis unit
e. Begin long-term psychodynamic psychotherapy

43. An 8-year-old white boy is brought to your office for evaluation of difficulties in the home and at school. His mother states that he is very difficult to manage at home. At school he seems to have difficulties following instructions, frequently forgets his homework, and often speaks out in class without having been called on. He has had psychological testing that demonstrates an above average IQ and no evidence of learning disability. Which of the following will be the most appropriate means to manage this boy?

a. Venlafaxine
b. Psychodynamic psychotherapy
c. Atomoxetine and behavioral therapy
d. Citalopram and cognitive therapy
e. Supportive psychotherapy
f. Haloperidol

44. A 4-year-old boy watches his father use a fork. The child then raises a fork and uses it in a similar fashion to feed himself. This is an example of:

a. Projection
b. Regression
c. Modeling
d. Classical conditioning
e. Operant conditioning

45. You have been called to evaluate a patient in the emergency department. The patient had been highly combative. He has a long history of schizoaffective disorder. The patient has been present for three emergency ward shifts. Initially, he was managed with several doses of intramuscular haloperidol. He appeared to respond but then began to demonstrate agitation that was then treated with oral olanzapine. The patient then became increasingly agitated and received high-dose intramuscular ziprasidone. The patient then became delirious with unstable blood pressure and diaphoresis, fever, rigidity, and then seizures. What is his likely diagnosis at this time?

a. Serotonin's syndrome
b. Neuroleptic malignant syndrome
c. Dystonia
d. Akathisia
e. Disulfiram-related toxicity

46. A college student presents with symptoms of depression. She states that she was doing very well up until 1 week previously. In fact, she states that she had not needed any sleep, her creativity was at an all-time high, and she was unbelievably productive in her work. She does report that she was uncharacteristically promiscuous. She states that this was followed by a period of irritability, difficulty concentrating, and a persistent inability to sleep. This was followed by the current depressive episode. Which of the following agents would be most appropriate for her maintenance therapy?

a. Venlafaxine
b. Mirtazapine
c. Lithium
d. Electroconvulsive therapy
e. Valium (diazepam)

47. A patient with treatment-refractory depression has received electroconvulsive therapy (ECT). Which of the following is true of this treatment?

a. Bilateral ECT has fewer side effects than unilateral
b. Bilateral ECT is more effective than unilateral
c. ECT is indicated only for refractory depression
d. The most common side effect is seizures
e. ECT is contraindicated in psychosis

48. An 85-year-old woman with no prior psychiatric history is evaluated in the emergency ward for odd behavior. According to the patient's family, she has been awake for 2 or 3 days with constant talking and activity. On examination, the patient is agitated, pacing the room, talking non-stop and not allowing you to interrupt her, and appears a bit paranoid. The most appropriate action is:

a. To treat the patient with a mood stabilizer for bipolar disorder
b. to treat the patient with synthetic thyroid hormone replacement
c. To treat the patient with an antidepressant medication
d. To order a thorough medical and neurological workup
e. To treat the patient with an antipsychotic medication for schizophrenia

49. A 72-year-old white man presents to the emergency ward after his daughter found him sitting on his bed with a loaded pistol in his hand. The patient denies depression or suicidal thinking and states that he was planning to clean the gun and that he keeps the gun for prowlers. The patient's daughter reports that he has seemed despondent

since his wife died a few months ago. He has lost a great deal of weight and has not been sleeping or grooming himself well. The most important initial management for this patient would include:

a. A nutritional consult
b. Psychiatric hospitalization
c. Outpatient psychotherapy referral
d. Outpatient psychopharmacology referral
e. Neurological consultation

50. Two elements of the above patient's history indicate that he is at increased risk for suicide. The first is major depression. The second is:

a. Weight loss
b. Lack of sleep
c. Hopelessness
d. Age, race, and gender
e. Poor grooming

51. Once hospitalized in a secure setting, appropriate treatments for this patient include:

a. Buspirone
b. Dialectical behavioral psychotherapy
c. Propanolol
d. Mirtazapine
e. Valproate

52. The patient is admitted to the hospital and treatment is initiated with mirtazapine. However, the patient continues to worsen and is unable to eat or drink. He continually ruminates about his hopelessness and desire to die. He has severe psychomotor retardation and has little spontaneous speech. A reasonable next step in treating this patient is:

a. Decrease the mirtazapine
b. Evaluate the patient for electroconvulsive therapy
c. Cognitive-behavioral therapy
d. Multivitamins
e. Add gabapentin

53. A 22-year-old man is brought to the local emergency ward by the police after being arrested in a grocery store for causing a disturbance. The nature of the disturbance is unclear, but the police indicate that the man was repeatedly accusing them of working for the National Security Agency and having a plan to "put him away." Upon examination, the young man appears agitated, disheveled, and frightened. He has been handcuffed to the bed by hospital security, and is straining at his restraints. His speech is quite pressured and he is very upset that you wish to measure his vital signs with the equipment in the room. He states "you are going to give me away." The most likely diagnosis at this point is:

a. Panic disorder
b. Heroin intoxication

c. Attention-deficit/hyperactivity disorder
d. Schizophrenia, paranoid subtype
e. Hypothyroidism

54. A 27-year-old man complains of excess sleepiness during the day and having intense dreams at times when he thinks he is still awake. He notes that he sometimes has an irresistible urge to sleep and has fallen asleep on multiple occasions even while driving. He feels refreshed after a daytime nap. Upon questioning, he reports that he sometimes has "drop" attacks characterized by sudden weakness in his whole body. He remains alert during the drop attacks but does fall to the floor. An appropriate treatment intervention is:

a. Continuous positive airway pressure at night to improve abnormal breathing during sleep
b. Administration of zoldipem (Ambien) at bedtime to improve nighttime sleep
c. Valproic acid to treat seizure activity
d. Modafinil to improve daytime alertness
e. Olanzapine to improve daytime alertness

55. A 57-year-old man with a past medical history of "liver problems" is seen in psychiatric consultation in the hospital intensive care unit because of agitation and confusion. The available history indicates that the patient was involved in a motor vehicle accident 72 hours ago in which he sustained a tibial fracture requiring surgical procedures for repair. The patient suffered no head injury or loss of consciousness during the accident. His medications since arriving in the hospital have included only antibiotics and opiate pain relievers. The diagnosis most consistent with agitation and confusion in this patient is:

a. Dementia
b. Psychotic disorder
c. Delirium
d. Antisocial personality disorder
e. Akathisia

56. The above patient's laboratory results include elevations in multiple liver enzymes with moderate anemia, leukopenia, and thrombocytopenia. A potentially critical treatment or diagnostic intervention at this point would include:

a. Transfusion of packed red blood cells
b. Evaluation for pulmonary embolism
c. Administration of an antidepressant medication
d. Administration of intravenous thiamine
e. Increase in the dosage of opiate pain reliever

57. Additional history obtained from the above patient's family indicates that he drinks alcohol on a daily basis. His minimum daily consumption of alcohol consists of a 12-pack of regular beer, but he often consumes more than twice that

amount. The patient's vital signs reveal a heart rate of 130 beats per minute and a blood pressure of 180/110 mm Hg. An additional critical treatment at this point would include:

a. Buspirone to treat withdrawal symptoms
b. Propanolol to treat hypertension and tachycardia
c. Intravenous hydration to treat tachycardia
d. A benzodiazepine to treat withdrawal symptoms
e. Clonidine to treat hypertension

58. The above patient responds to treatment and his confusion and autonomic instability resolve. He is successfully tapered from benzodiazepines and has not required opiate pain relievers for the past 7 days. He expresses a desire to stop drinking alcohol and requests treatment for alcohol dependence. An appropriate pharmacological intervention might include:

a. An antidepressant medication of the selective serotonin-reuptake inhibitor class
b. A benzodiazepine medication
c. An antihypertensive medication
d. An opiate analgesic medication
e. Naltrexone

59. A 12-year-old girl presents with her foster mother for a routine pediatric visit. The girl seems quiet and she does not make eye contact with you as you enter the room. Her foster mother says that she has been having difficulties socially in school. She has trouble making friends and often has conflicts with classmates. She has trouble seeing the "big picture" of problems that face her and she often gets lost in the details of projects that she is assigned. She is awkward in her interactions. Her foster mother says that she can be quite verbally articulate and writes extremely well. You query her for depressive or psychotic symptoms and she denies either. Once you ask her about one of her projects she tells you about the intricacies of building a radio from scratch. She engages with you briefly but still appears uncomfortable. She denies any significant anxiety. The most likely diagnosis is:

a. Asperger's syndrome
b. Autism
c. Avoidant personality disorder
d. Anxiety disorder not otherwise specified
e. Posttraumatic stress disorder

60. An 87-year-old woman with a history of mild mixed dementia is admitted for confusion and a urinary tract infection. When the nurse attempts to place a Foley catheter to improve urine drainage, the patient becomes agitated and refuses the catheter. The medical team requests that the psychiatric consultant assess the patient's ability to consent to medical procedures. On exam, the patient is alert and oriented to person, place,

date, and time. The consultant explains in detail the reason the catheter is indicated and the medical consequences of failing to receive appropriate treatment. The patient states, "I don't want a catheter." Which element of Informed Consent has this patient satisfied?

a. Consent
b. Information
c. Concrete logic
d. Duty
e. Capacity

61. You are working in an outpatient psychotherapy clinic when your patient tells you that she plans to kill her landlord. The patient calls the landlord by name, and mentions that he lives just down the street from her. You tell the patient that you are quite concerned about these homicidal feelings and recommend inpatient psychiatric admission. Before you can react, the patient bolts from the office and escapes. You realize that you must attempt to warn the patient's landlord about the patient's statements. Your actions are grounded in which of the following legal precedents?

a. The *Tarasoff* decision
b. The M'Naghten rule
c. *Griswold v. Connecticut*
d. Swedish Common Law
e. Negligence

62. A 29-year-old man is dropped off by friends at the emergency ward. The patient complains of chest pain. On examination the patient is nervous, diaphoretic, and pacing. His vital signs indicate a heart rate of 132 with a blood pressure of 175/100. The patient is afebrile. An electrocardiogram reveals sinus tachycardia with ST segment depressions in the anterior leads. The patient smokes 1.5 packs per day of cigarettes. He does not recall a prior diagnosis of hypertension, hypercholesterolemia, or diabetes. He has no known prior history of "heart trouble." He denies alcohol or drug use. A critical diagnostic test at this point is:

a. Abdominal ultrasound
b. Electroencephalogram
c. Urine drug screen
d. Hematocrit
e. Liver function tests

63. A urine test obtained on the above patient reveals cocaine and cocaine metabolites in the urine specimen. The patient has a mild myocardial infarction without significant arrhythmia or other complications. Upon confrontation, he states that he rarely uses cocaine and this was the first time in many months. However, upon checking the patient's chart from prior visits, it is clear that the patient has had several emergency ward visits for chest pain with cocaine-positive urine tests over the last year. At this point, you can make the following diagnosis with confidence:

a. Polydrug abuse
b. Antisocial personality disorder
c. Cocaine dependence
d. Myocardial infarction
e. Malingering

64. A 57-year-old man with a history of chronic alcoholism is placed in a nursing home for alcohol-related amnestic disorder. This condition is associated with damage to the following brain regions:
a. The brainstem and frontal lobes
b. The hippocampus, fornix, and mammillary bodies
c. The thalamus and cingulate gyrus
d. The caudate and putamen
e. The cerebellum

65. A 25-year-old female has episodes of recurrent, unexpected anxiety, with palpitations, diaphoresis, chest pain, and a fear of losing control. She avoids socializing and shopping due to fear of recurrence of these episodes. Alterations in the following neurotransmitter system are strongly linked to this disorder:
a. Glycine
b. Melatonin
c. Substance P
d. Enkephalin
e. GABA

66. An 11-year-old boy presents in your outpatient clinic with his father for a routine visit. The father says the child is developing well. He began playing soccer 2 years ago. The father said that he is sometimes a "sore loser," and other times he is pleased with the scores that he achieves. He sometimes thinks he is "useless" if he doesn't score at a game. The father said that he praises him whether he scores or not and tries to teach him new techniques for improving his game when they play together on the weekends. The son tells you that he feels like he is a good player and only sometimes thinks that he is the worst player on the team. According to Erikson's life cycle stages, the boy is dealing with what developmental conflict?
a. Intimacy versus isolation
b. Identity versus role confusion
c. Initiative versus guilt
d. Industry versus inferiority
e. Ego integrity versus despair

67. A 24-year-old woman presents in the emergency department complaining that her nose is crooked. She is examined by you and you find no evidence that it is abnormal. She pulls out a mirror and looks at herself. "See," pointing to her nose, "Don't you see how ugly it is?" She tells you that she cannot continue walking around in public with this nose. She feels that everyone notices it and has gone to a number of plastic surgeons to try to get it corrected. None has been willing to operate on her nose to fix it. You ask a colleague to examine the patient, and she draws the same conclusion as you. The patient has:
a. Body dysmorphic disorder
b. Exhibitionism
c. Borderline personality disorder
d. Social phobia
e. Posttraumatic stress disorder

68. A 50-year-old man is brought to your office by his family. He states that he is doing fine and that he has no memory trouble. The family, however, states that the patient has become apathetic, inconsiderate, and neglects his personal care. He has documented mild memory difficulty. He has no history of coronary artery disease or hypertension. A workup to date has included thiamine, vitamin B_{12}, folate, niacin levels, all of which were normal. An HIV test was negative. A head CT scan with and without contrast demonstrated frontal and temporal atrophy. What is your diagnosis?
a. Alzheimer's disease
b. Pick's disease
c. Huntington's chorea
d. Vascular dementia
e. Creutzfeldt–Jakob

69. A 46-year-old woman presents to you for an initial psychiatric evaluation. She has had long-standing problems with mood and significant difficulties with interpersonal relationships. She tells you that she was in psychotherapy for 5 years with a doctor from another city. She met with him several times a week and describes talking with him about her early childhood, her relationships with her parents, and subsequent relationships with important people in her life. In the end, she felt that she understood herself a lot better and could have better relationships, but her mood has remained a problem. The patient was likely undergoing what kind of treatment?
a. Cognitive-behavioral therapy
b. Psychoanalytic psychotherapy
c. Interpersonal therapy
d. Behavior therapy
e. Dialectical behavioral therapy

70. A 57-year-old man from out of town sees you in walk-in clinic to obtain replacement prescriptions because his original prescriptions have been lost. He explains to you that he is a recovering alcoholic with depression and anxiety. In addition to paroxetine, he is prescribed a medication that his doctor at home said would decrease his cravings for alcohol. He can't recall the name of the medication but he did drink a large amount of alcohol one time since he has been on it and did not feel ill. He thinks the medicine

may have worked because he lost interest in continuing drinking the next day and has not relapsed since. The medication is most likely to be:
a. Disulfiram
b. Zolpidem
c. Buspirone
d. Naltrexone
e. Metoclopromide

71. A 45-year-old alcoholic man with hepatic cirrhosis is admitted for alcohol detoxification. The attending physician on-call instructs you to treat the patient with routine treatment including thiamine, folate, and benzodiazepines. She tells you that, since the patient likely has impaired hepatic metabolism, you should choose a benzodiazepine that is metabolized by conjugation and that doesn't have long-acting metabolites. A reasonable choice is:
a. Oxazepam
b. Diazepam
c. Chlordiazepoxide
d. Buspirone
e. Clonazepam

72. A 73-year-old man is admitted to the hospital for lobar pneumonia and develops delirium. In thinking about delirium, you remember that dementia is a risk factor for the future development of delirium. In reviewing this patient's history, you learn that he has a 40-pack-year history of cigarette smoking, hypercholesterolemia, hypertension, type 2 diabetes mellitus, and coronary artery disease. This patient has known risk factors primarily for what type of dementia?
a. Huntington's-related dementia
b. Vascular-related dementia
c. Jacob–Creutzfeldt-related dementia
d. Parkinson's-related dementia
e. HIV-related dementia

73. A 23-year-old man seeks psychological counseling because he is worried that he isn't "normal." After learning a bit about the patient, you ask him to tell you what he needs help with. The patient states that he thinks his sex drive is much lower than that of his peers. He reports that he rarely has a sexual fantasy and almost never has an interest in sex. This patient has a disturbance in what phase of the sexual response cycle?
a. Excitement
b. Desire
c. Resolution
d. Orgasm
e. Plateau

74. A 56-year-old man with a history of mild hypertension and obesity presents to his primary care physician for treatment of daytime sleepiness and fatigue. The patient reports that he has been getting progressively more fatigued over the past 2 to 3 years and has gained around 25 lb because he has no energy to move around. He has been increasing his caffeine intake to the point that he feels jittery and nervous, but is still tired, dozes off quite frequently during the day, and has fairly frequent headaches. After obtaining a detailed medical and psychiatric history, you ask the patient about his time in bed at night. He states that he sleeps alone after his last bed-partner complained that he snored very loudly and sounded like he was choking all night. After completing the interview, you make the following provisional diagnosis for the patient's complaints:
a. Hypothyroidism
b. Hyperthyroidism
c. Hypochondriasis
d. Major depression
e. Sleep-related breathing disorder
f. Narcolepsy

75. As an emergency department triage officer you have been asked to develop a protocol for admissions. While it is understood that any patient might necessitate admission, some conditions are generally self-limited. A patient in withdrawal from which of the following medications would most likely necessitate admission?
a. Crack cocaine
b. Crystal methamphetamine
c. Marijuana
d. Barbiturates
e. Nicotine

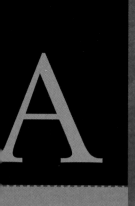

A Answers

1. d (Chapter 18)

Malpractice requires the presence of four elements: negligence, duty, direct causation, and damages. Negligence includes failing to meet the standard of care.

2. b (Chapter 15)

The patient described is experiencing extrapyramidal symptoms. The first line of treatment for the symptoms is an anticholinergic agent. Of all the agents listed only benztropine is primarily an anticholinergic medication. Methylphenidate and pemoline are both psychostimulants. Atenolol is a beta-blocker and may be used to manage blood pressure, to treat akathisia (another side effect of psychotropic medications), and other conditions. Clonidine is primarily used as an antihypertensive and is effective in the treatment of opiate withdrawal, attention-deficit disorder, and Tourette's syndrome.

3. a (Chapter 9)

Somatization disorder is characterized by multiple chronic medical complaints that include pain, gastrointestinal disturbances, sexual symptoms, and pseudoneurologic symptoms that are not due to a medical illness. The diagnosis of somatization disorder can be challenging because it requires the presence of (i) four pain symptoms at different sites or in different bodily functions, (ii) two gastrointestinal symptoms, (iii) at least one sexual symptom (not sexual pain), and (iv) one pseudoneurological symptom. The history of physical complaints must start before age 30. Conversion disorder involves complaints of sensory or motor dysfunction that are not due to neurologic dysfunction. Pain disorder is suspected when psychological factors play a major role in mediating expression and impact of pain. Hypochondriasis is characterized by a preoccupation with having serious disease based on a misinterpretation of bodily function and sensation. Body dysmorphic disorder is characterized by excessive concern with a perceived defect in appearance.

4. c (Chapters 7 and 9)

The child is likely experiencing sleep terror disorder that occurs during delta sleep. Stage 0 is awake. Non-rapid-eye-movement (NREM) sleep includes stages 1, 2, 3, and 4. Delta sleep is a subdivision of NREM sleep comprising stages 3 and 4. Nightmares generally occur during REM sleep.

5. d (Chapter 3)

The symptoms described are consistent with a panic attack. The technique described cognitive-behavioral therapy. Subsequently the patient will learn that the sensations are innocuous and self-limited, which generally diminishes the panicky response. Exposure therapy involves incrementally confronting a feared stimulus. Classical conditioning is a form of learning in which a neutral stimulus is repetitively paired with a natural stimulus with the result that the previously neutral stimulus alone then becomes capable of eliciting the same response as the natural stimulus.

6. a (Chapters 12 and 14)

Alprazolam is a benzodiazepine and acts at the GABA receptor. Mirtazapine blocks the alpha-2-reuptake receptor as well as having postsynaptic activity. Imipramine is a tricyclic antidepressant and acts by blocking presynaptic reuptake of serotonin and norepinephrine. Paroxetine is a selective serotonin-reuptake inhibitor. Phenelzine is a monoamine oxidase inhibitor that blocks the presynaptic enzymes that catabolize norepinephrine, dopamine, and serotonin.

7. a (Chapter 6)

The patient is likely inducing vomiting mechanically with her right index finger. This has resulted in hypokalemia, which has produced the characteristic electrocardiographic findings and cardiac arrhythmia. Esophageal rupture is also a possible complication of induced vomiting. Patients with bulimia nervosa may maintain near normal body weights.

8. d (Chapter 15)

Donepezil and tacrine both reversibly bind the enzyme acetyl-cholinesterase. This reduces the enzymes activity, which is to hydrolyze acetylcholine in the synapse. Reducing the activity of acetylcholinesterase is thought to raise the presynaptic concentration of acetylcholine released by axons of the remaining cholinergic neurons. Initially, these drugs reduce cognitive impairment; however, this effect wanes with the progressive loss of cholinergic neurons that is seen in this disease.

9. d (Chapter 1)

The patient presents with seizure that is most likely due to acute hyponatremia. The hyponatremia could have many causes. The syndrome of inappropriate anti-diuretic hormone secretion or SIADH, which is often associated with oat cell carcinoma of the lung, is an unlikely cause of the hyponatremia in a non-smoker with a normal chest x-ray. Clozapine can cause seizures and may be a contributing factor to the seizure but would not cause hyponatremia. Hypertension can lead to cerebral dysfunction, but not usually seizures. This level of mild hypertension would not have neurologic effects. Serotonin's syndrome can cause confusion but does not cause seizures or hyponatremia. The diagnosis of exclusion would likely be polydipsia and is suggested by the staff person reporting her excessive cola drinking.

10. c (Chapter 4)

This patient shows many of the common features of borderline personality disorder. She displays maladaptive coping patterns to routine stress, emotional lability, perceives that she has been abandoned by the nurse, and self-injurious behavior. Although patients with this disorder have high rates of depression, she does not meet criteria for an episode currently. Although she displays some self-centeredness in her perception of the clinical staff interaction, the major issue is that she perceived being abandoned by the nurse. She undoubtedly experiences anxiety related to her maladaptive coping style, but does not provide evidence of a persistent pattern of worrying that would characterize generalized anxiety disorder. Finally, the self-injurious behavior of cutting or scratching her thighs would not constitute masochism as the patient does not experience sexual gratification from the behavior but rather a relief of emotional distress.

11. d (Chapter 4)

This man exhibits some common signs of narcissistic personality disorder. His disregard of the time of the appointment, grandiosity about his capabilities despite several failed jobs, and his sensitivity to a mild suggestion that he might have a problem are behaviors seen commonly with this disorder. Humiliation followed by anger is also a common manifestation of narcissistic personality. The condition can be quite disabling as a consequence of the difficulties such individuals have tolerating the perceived slights omnipresent in nearly every job setting. The aloofness and grandiosity are off-putting and diminish empathy from others for one's underlying pain. His interest in interacting and pursuing work relationships makes schizoid personality disorder unlikely. Although he is grandiose, his admission of inadequacy is not consistent with a persistent, delusional grandiosity. He is not self-destructive, impulsive, or afraid of abandonment, making borderline personality disorder unlikely. He exhibits no features of dependent personality disorder (extreme neediness and reliance on others for emotional support and decision making).

12. b (Chapter 3)

This patient has untreated panic disorder with a relatively late onset of the disorder. She has a family history of agoraphobia, a complication of panic disorder that this patient has developed. Her clinical history is not consistent with major depression. Her anxiety comes in classic waves of panic, not the constant worrying of a person with generalized anxiety. She has neither the specific fear of spiders necessary to diagnose arachnophobia nor the obsessions and compulsions of obsessive-compulsive disorder.

13. e (Chapters 7 and 15)

The child has developed symptoms of mania and psychosis while in the first few months of dextro-amphetamine therapy for a presumed case of attention-deficit disorder. The violence clearly warrants a hospitalization. What is unclear, especially given the extensive family history, is whether the symptoms are solely due to treatment or if the patient is having an initial episode of bipolar disorder or schizophrenia. The diagnosis is unclear, but the first thing that should be done is discontinuation of the dextro-amphetamine. Further treatment might include either an antipsychotic or a mood stabilizer. An antidepressant would be contraindicated in a patient without depression or anxiety who may be having a manic or psychotic episode. Group therapy would be helpful after the acute stabilization, but is not the first step in management.

14. d (Chapter 7)

The girl exhibits selective mutism. Commonly, children with this condition will speak normally at home but become mute at school. It is believed to be a childhood form of social anxiety disorder. While this selectively mute child might be depressed, her activity outside of school suggests otherwise. She and her family and teachers should be queried about the possibility of a school-related abuse situation leading to posttraumatic stress disorder, but we have no evidence of this currently. Children with autism fail to relate in all contexts, not just at school. Abulia is a neurological condition that results in a lack of affective expression. Children with selective mutism can be treated with a social group and antidepressant medication targeting their social anxiety. Some children will go on to develop social anxiety disorder or depression in later life.

15. e (Chapters 5 and 15)

The patient has opiate dependence and is most likely suffering from an opiate overdose. The initial symptoms of lacrimation, dilated pupils, piloerection, mild fever, and mild tachycardia are consistent with opiate withdrawal. The laboratory test you ordered was a urine drug screen that was positive for opiate metabolites. After confrontation during the initial visit, the patient confessed that she had sought opiate prescriptions from multiple physicians and had also been stealing narcotics from the hospital by pretending to give them to patients and then pocketing them. You had prescribed an inpatient admission for opiate detoxification followed by outpatient psychotherapy and self-help group involvement. The patient had successfully detoxified prior to being found unresponsive. Of the listed treatments, flumazenil is a benzodiazepine antagonist. Physostigmine is helpful in treating anticholinergic toxicity. Clonidine may help with symptoms of opiate withdrawal but not with opiate intoxication. Acamprosate is useful in the treatment of alcoholism. Naloxone is an opiate antagonist that can be life-saving in cases of opiate overdose. Alprazolam is a benzodiazepine that is useful in alcohol withdrawal. Thiamine and glucose are important treatments in patients who are found unresponsive and would also be important in the management of this patient in case other factors were contributing to the diagnosis.

16. c (Chapter 7)

This child has mental retardation. It falls in the mild range and the child should be educable but will require a special education curriculum. If his IQ was less than 50 but more than 30, he would have moderate mental retardation; whereas if it were 20 to 30, the retardation would be severe. He does not appear to have autism because he is able to communicate and makes eye contact. Finally, children with Asperger's disorder have either a normal or a high IQ and have awkward social skills with poor eye contact. Before finalizing this diagnosis, it would be important to rule out all potential medical causes for his poor intellectual function.

17. b (Chapter 10)

Suspected cases of elder abuse need to be reported to social services. Sending the patient home and arranging for outpatient follow-up leaves the patient at significant risk and violates mandated reporting laws in many states. Although it may be tempting to confront the suspected perpetrators, it is generally better to leave this in the hands of experienced social workers who can sort out the social situation and report the appropriate persons to authorities. A reporting physician may be sued by the accused abusers, but risk management should be called only after social services have consulted on the case.

18. c (Chapter 10)

Patients suffering from abuse sometimes appear for treatment with their abusers. This couple may have alcoholism, given the presence of an alcohol smell on their breath without evidence of intoxication, a potential sign of high alcohol tolerance. Your primary fiduciary responsibility is to your patient. Abused people may be afraid to confront their abusers due to fear of retaliation. Therefore, it would not be appropriate to call the police or to confront the suspected abuser without more information. If you try to get more information with the alleged abuser present, you may arouse suspicion in the abuser who may then take the abused patient and leave. Finally, calling around in an investigative mode violates patient confidentiality and is outside the role of a physician treating a patient. The best option is to find a tactful way to speak with the patient alone to ask about potential abuse. With this approach, you preserve your patient's right to privacy, do not risk your intervention resulting in more harm to the patient, and provide a safe opportunity for the patient to seek help from a physician.

19. b (Chapter 11)

The patient is rigid, akinetic, hyperpyrexic, and unresponsive with an elevated CPK. This is neuroleptic malignant syndrome (NMS) until proven otherwise. Serotonin's syndrome should be thought of but the characteristic symptoms of shivering, hyperreflexia, clonus, and gastrointestinal symptoms are not present. Muscular rigidity commonly suggests NMS, but can develop in severe cases of serotonin's syndrome. Tardive dyskinesia is not associated with fever and akinesis. A dystonia would be localized to one or two muscle groups and would not cause the systemic signs. Pneumonia would cause the systemic signs but not the focal neurological signs.

20. e (Chapters 2 and 13)

The patient shows classic symptoms of mania: Rapid speech, grandiosity, decreased need for sleep, and spending sprees. Of the medicines listed, valproic acid, an anticonvulsant mood stabilizer, would be the most helpful. Flumazenil, a benzodiazepine antagonist would not have any impact. Fluoxetine would not treat the mania and may, in fact, worsen it. Acamprosate counteracts alcohol dependence but does not improve mania. Gabapentin, while initially suspected of having mood-stabilizing properties, does not treat mania and would be less effective than standard treatments such as valproic acid.

21. a (Chapter 7)

This child displays the classic diagnostic criterion for autism, namely: (i) impaired social interactions; (ii) impaired communication; and (iii) stereotyped behavior or interests. The child does not display evidence of a formal thought disorder or ongoing psychosis, so would not meet criteria for schizophrenia. Conduct disorder is a behavioral disturbance where a child violates the basic rights of others and does not adhere to rules and societal norms. It is the childhood equivalent of antisocial personality disorder in adults. Attention-deficit disorder is characterized by a persistent attention disturbance in at least two different settings (such as school and home). It may be accompanied by hyperactivity, in which circumstance attention-deficit/hyperactivity disorder would be diagnosed. Separation anxiety disorder is characterized by anxiety as evidenced by behavioral disturbance (such as crying) when separated from a primary caregiver.

22. e (Chapter 10)

Among all the factors listed, hopelessness has been shown to be one of the most reliable indicators of long-term suicide risk. Major depression and other mood disorders and substance abuse disorders are also risk factors for suicide.

23. c (Chapter 11)

The patient has moderate granulocytopenia. Although many medications can cause granulocytopenia or agranulocytosis, clozapine carries the highest risk of all the antipsychotics for this major adverse drug reaction. It is also the only antipsychotic agent that requires frequent white blood cell monitoring.

24. b (Chapter 5)

This patient appears to have a profound yearning for connection and a dependent relationship with his elderly mother. He overly depends on his mother to steer his life, including making minor decisions. He likely fears abandonment by the mother on whom he depends, but he differs from those with borderline personality disorder in that he has a more stable sense of self and is not impulsive and self-destructive. His self-esteem is not impaired and he lacks the grandiosity that would be seen in a person with narcissistic personality. Although the patient works in an often solitary job, he is not an aloof, detached loner with schizoid personality disorder. Also, there is no evidence of the magical thinking that would characterize schizotypal personality disorder.

25. a (Chapter 1)

A diagnosis of schizophrenia requires a greater than 6-month period of positive and negative symptoms of psychosis combined with social and occupational deterioration. Bipolar disorder requires the presence of at least one episode of mania and usually consists of cycles of mania and depression. Psychosis is common in the manic phase of bipolar illness, but this patient does not display symptoms of mania (i.e., pressured speech, decreased sleep, increased energy, etc.). Major depression may be associated with psychosis, but this patient does not provide evidence of having major depression. Alcohol abuse can lead to psychosis, especially auditory hallucinosis, but other symptoms of alcohol abuse would be present. Paranoid personality disorder does not lead to the level of severe social and occupational dysfunction experienced by this patient.

26. e (Chapter 4)

This patient exhibits a pervasive pattern of flagrant disregard for the rules and laws of society. A childhood history of severe neglect or abuse is not uncommon. Despite the report of a childhood trauma, a diagnosis of posttraumatic stress disorder is not made unless there is hyperarousal, intrusive recollection of the trauma, and efforts to avoid recollection of the trauma. His denial of mood disturbance and lack of either prior hospitalizations or family history makes both bipolar disorder and cyclothymic disorder unlikely. This patient may have been diagnosed with conduct disorder in childhood. When conduct disorder behavior persists into adulthood, the diagnosis becomes antisocial personality disorder.

27. c (Chapter 16)

This patient exhibits the classic symptoms of akathisia, a common side effect of antipsychotic medications. Patients with this side effect exhibit agitation, restlessness, and pacing. They usually endorse an inner feeling of restlessness (often localized to the legs). It is important to distinguish akathisia from restlessness and agitation due to worsening psychosis or anxiety. Other movement disorders, such as dystonia (muscle spasm), tardive dyskinesia (slow, involuntary muscle movements), or parkinsonism (pill-rolling tremor, festinating gait, masked facies), should always be ruled out in patients taking neuroleptics. Patients with neuroleptic malignant syndrome can present with agitation or motor excitability, but the absence of fever and a normal serum CPK make this diagnosis unlikely.

28. d (Chapter 7)

Tourette's disorder is characterized by involuntary vocal and motor tics. Sometimes the vocal tics are grunts or barks, but they can develop into word tics. Tourette's disorder is more common in young males (3:1 male–female ratio) and onset is usually in late adolescence. Adolescent rebellion is a colloquial term for certain types of teenage behavior but does not explain vocal and motor tics. Schizophrenia is not likely because this young man does not have psychotic symptoms. Substance abuse can produce a behavioral change in an individual, but vocal and motor tics are not classic. Conduct disorder is diagnosed when a child consistently violates the basic rights of others and ignores societal rules and norms. A child suspected of having Tourette's disorder should have a careful medical and neurologic evaluation. Wilson's disease and Huntington's disease both present with movement disturbance that could be confused with motor tics and therefore need to be ruled out, and an electroencephalogram should be performed to assess for seizure disorder.

29. a (Chapters 13 and 16)

Since lithium is renally cleared, its serum level can be affected by states of dehydration or renal insufficiency. Signs of lithium toxicity, including coarse tremor, confusion, ataxia, and diarrhea, are evident in this patient. Although oxcarbazepine toxicity can similarly result in ataxia and confusion, it is not associated with coarse tremor or diarrhea. Oxcarbazepine levels are also not as sensitive to levels of dehydration. Fluoxetine can cause nausea, headache, restlessness, insomnia, and anorgasmia. It is generally nontoxic even in overdose. Serotonin's syndrome can cause tremor and confusion but not ataxia.

30. a (Chapters 1 and 2)

This patient presents with psychotic symptoms and agitation. Until further history is obtained or future episodes are observed, the diagnosis is uncertain. This could be a so-called "first break" of schizophreniform disorder that may persist for the required 6 months to meet the criteria for schizophrenia. It might be a manic episode with psychotic features in a patient with underlying bipolar disorder or schizoaffective disorder. The psychosis may also be substance-induced (e.g., amphetamine-induced psychotic disorder). Although patients with generalized anxiety disorder can present with restlessness or irritability, they are usually not agitated and do not have auditory hallucinations or thought disorder. Patients with winter depression and atypical depression usually present with symptoms of decreased energy, increased appetite, and increased sleep. They also complain of psychomotor slowing. Individuals with obsessive-compulsive disorder have unreasonable obsessions and compulsions.

31. e (Chapters 2, 5, and 10)

The described vignette is commonly seen in patients who attempt suicide. To accept the patient's assertion that the event was accidental would be inappropriate in the face of a life-threatening event. Patients often attempt suicide and then deny any intention to self-harm. Intoxication with alcohol or other drugs is not uncommon. A head CT does not appear clinically indicated unless one suspects head injury or intracranial process predisposing to self-injurious behavior. A thyroid-stimulating hormone level might be appropriate if the patient is found to have depression. The patient may have alcohol dependence or abuse warranting a referral to Alcoholics Anonymous, but the available history does not support such a diagnosis at this point. Obtaining additional history is critical for properly evaluating this patient. In such cases, collateral history of prior suicidal statements to family or friends is often uncovered. Or, behavioral change consistent with a diagnosis of depression may be found. Denial or ambivalence regarded suicide attempts is frequently present.

32. b (Chapters 2, 5, and 10)

Forming a treatment alliance with the patient is the best path to obtaining additional information from him and helping him gain insight into his circumstances. In the clinical setting, it is often unclear whether patients who attempt and then deny self-injury in the context of clear psychosocial stress and vocational and interpersonal difficulties are conscious of their suicidal intentions. But, denial of suicide attempts is quite common and the use of intoxicants prior to such attempts is also a common clinical scenario. A discussion of alcohol use and misuse is also important, but the most urgent medical consideration at the point is suicidality. An antidepressant would be indicated if additional history supported the diagnosis of major depression.

33. b (Chapters 12 and 16)

Akathisia is most commonly caused by antipsychotic medications, particularly typical antipsychotics (neuroleptics). Akathisia produced by drugs in the selective serotonin-reuptake inhibitor class is less likely, but these medications are so widely used and are prescribed by so many nonpsychiatric physicians that this important side effect may be misdiagnosed. Akathisia is profoundly distressing to some patients, and in some cases leads to attempted or successful suicide. It is easily treatable by removing the offending agent in most cases. Adding beta-blockers and benzodiazepines is also helpful.

34. c (Chapters 13 and 16)

The best explanation for the patient's condition at the moment is drug toxicity due to elevated carbamazepine levels. The patient displays known symptoms consistent with carbamazepine toxicity. The clue to making the diagnosis rests with the sequence of events. The patient likely was noncompliant with his medications as an outpatient leading to reduced levels of mood stabilizer and a manic break. Upon admission, he was restarted at his usual outpatient doses, which presumably provide a therapeutic drug level when taken as scheduled. Then, an antibiotic is added. We are not provided with the name of the drug, but it is important to remember that some antibiotics, such as macrolide antibiotics, may inhibit the metabolism of medications metabolized by the liver's cytochrome p450 enzyme system.

35. a (Chapter 1)

Catatonic schizophrenia requires the presence of catatonic symptoms (motor and vocal changes). Disorganized schizophrenia requires the presence of disorganized speech and behavior and inappropriate affect. Undifferentiated schizophrenia is diagnosed when criteria are not met for another subtype. Residual schizophrenia is diagnosed when a patient who formerly had prominent positive symptoms of schizophrenia now has only residual negative symptoms or minor positive symptoms.

36. e (Chapters 1 and 16)

The patient has developed neuroleptic-induced parkinsonism (also known as pseudo-parkinsonism), a drug-induced condition resembling Parkinson's disease. The "pill rolling" tremor, festinating gait, and difficulty initiating movements are all symptoms of Parkinson's disease. Since the disease is due to low cerebral dopamine levels, drugs that block dopamine receptors are most likely to mimic the disease. Neither lorazepam nor benztropine block dopamine receptors. Quetiapine and clozapine both block dopamine receptors, but they only weakly block dopamine receptors and are less likely to cause pseudo-parkinsonism. Haloperidol, a potent dopamine blocker, is most likely to cause the syndrome.

37. a (Chapters 5 and 8)

Continue his current treatment regimen with downward adjustments in opiate and benzodiazepine dosing as pain and alcohol withdrawal symptoms subside. Gradual taper of opiate pain medication with clinical improvement and gradual taper of benzodiazepines with improved symptoms of alcohol withdrawal are the appropriate treatment at this point. Naltrexone is indicated for treating alcohol dependence but should not be given to a person taking opiates because it may precipitate severe withdrawal. Judicious use of opiates is necessary in many drug- or alcohol-dependent individuals in circumstances normally requiring treatment with opiate medications. Benzodiazepines, although potentially addictive, are used for the short-term treatment of alcohol withdrawal symptoms and should be slowly tapered to avoid precipitating a seizure or other severe withdrawal symptoms. Antidepressant medications may be useful in individuals with alcohol dependence and depression, but we are not provided with evidence of depression in this patient.

38. a (Chapters 5 and 15)

Following successful alcohol detoxification, combined treatment with Alcohol Anonymous (AA), cognitive-behavioral therapy (CBT), and pharmacological management with naltrexone or acamprosate is indicated. Naltrexone, CBT, AA, or acamprosate alone would also be useful treatments but are not as effective individually as is combination therapy. The exact mechanism of naltrexone in preventing or lessening the severity of alcohol relapse is unknown but is presumably related to the action of naltrexone as a mu opioid antagonist. Acamprosate may work via numerous mechanisms, including as a modulator of glutamate function. Duloxetine is an antidepressant that might be used in treating the patient if he had major depression. Oxazepam is used for acute detoxification for alcohol dependence but is contraindicated after detoxification as it may precipitate relapse or lead to oxazepam abuse or dependence in alcoholism.

39. c (Chapters 2 and 12)

The patient has likely developed substance-induced mania caused by fluoxetine treatment for her postpartum depression. This is particularly common in postpartum patients treated with antidepressants. The most appropriate treatment would be to stop fluoxetine and begin a mood stabilizer. Electroconvulsive therapy can be used for both depression and mania, but only in very severe cases that are refractory to other treatment. Dialectical behavioral therapy is indicated for borderline personality disorder. Cognitive-behavioral therapy examines cognitive distortions and is primarily useful for depression and anxiety disorders.

40. e (Chapters 1 and 18)

This clinical scenario would be considered a true emergency and performing a tracheotomy to stabilize the patient's airway would not require informed consent. Commitment is not necessary or appropriate in this circumstance. However, committed patients also do not require informed consent for treatment. If this were not an emergency situation, each of the other issues would be a valid concern.

41. e (Chapters 2 and 12)

The patient's symptoms are consistent with major depression. Selective serotonin-reuptake inhibitors are a first-line choice for the treatment of depression, but sexual side effects are common and could potentially further complicate his relationship with his wife. Tricyclic antidepressants are very effective but are generally considered second-line antidepressants due to their toxicity and side-effect profiles. Lithium is primarily an augmentative treatment for depression. Although very effective, monoamine oxidase inhibitors (MAOIs) are not used as first-line antidepressant treatments due to their requirement for dietary restrictions. The dietary limitations of MAOIs would additionally limit their usefulness in a patient who works as a chef. Electroconvulsive therapy is not contraindicated 3 months after myocardial infarction, but is indicated only for severe or refractory depression.

42. c (Chapters 4 and 17)

The patient described has borderline personality disorder. Dialectical behavioral therapy was developed specifically for the treatment of borderline personality disorder. Patients with borderline personality disorder often require adjunctive treatments for their substance abuse, mood disorders, and other comorbidities. Because of their primitive defenses, they are generally not good candidates for long-term psychodynamic psychotherapy.

43. c (Chapters 7 and 15)

The child described above meets the criteria for attention-deficit/hyperactivity disorder, which is generally managed with psychostimulants. Methylphenidate is the first-line agent followed by D-amphetamine. These are sometimes avoided because of bizarre behavior or long-term physical effects such as weight loss and inhibited body growth. Alternatively, children can be treated with atomoxetine. Behavioral management is also one of the mainstays of treatment.

44. c (Chapter 17)

Modeling is learning based on observing others and mimicking their actions. Classical conditioning is learning where a neutral stimulus is paired with a natural stimulus, with the result that the previously neutral stimulus alone becomes capable of eliciting the same response as the natural stimulus. Operant conditioning is a form of learning in which environmental events influence the acquisition of new behaviors or the extinction of existing behaviors. Projection and regression are both defense mechanisms.

45. b (Chapters 1, 11, and 16)

Neuroleptic malignant syndrome (NMS) can occur at any time during the use of antipsychotic medications. It is most frequently seen during periods of dehydration or rapid escalation of dose. Serotonin's syndrome can present similarly to NMS but usually has less muscular rigidity. Dystonia is a neuroleptic-induced movement disorder characterized by muscle spasms. Akathisia consists of a subjective sensation of inner restlessness or a strong desire to move one's body. Disulfiram serves to prevent alcohol ingestion through the fear of the consequences of its interaction with the metabolism of alcohol. Disulfiram blocks the oxidation of the acetaldehyde, which leads to flushing, headache, sweating, dry mouth, nausea, vomiting, and dizziness.

46. c (Chapters 2, 12, and 13)

The patient described meets probable criteria for bipolar disorder. Mood stabilizers and antipsychotic medications are the mainstays of maintenance therapy. Benzodiazepines may be used also in the management of acute mania. Antidepressants should be used with caution because of the possibility of inducing mania or producing a more severe mania.

47. b (Chapter 12)

The most common side effect of electroconvulsive therapy (ECT) is short-term memory loss and confusion. Bilateral ECT is more effective than unilateral ECT but produces more cognitive side effects. ECT has some efficacy in refractory mania and in psychoses with prominent mood components or catatonia.

48. d (Chapters 1, 2, and 8)

This patient displays the key symptoms necessary for the diagnosis of an acute manic episode. However, the onset of bipolar disorder in someone of this age group with no prior psychiatric history is unlikely. Therefore, medical and neurological causes of the patient's behavioral change should be carefully assessed. A mood stabilizer or antipsychotic medication may be needed now or at a later point for symptom control, but would not be started for the specified diagnoses until a definitive workup is completed. An antidepressant would not help treat this symptom complex and might make the condition worse. The patient does have symptoms consistent with hyperthyroidism, but the treatment would not be to add more thyroid hormone.

49. b (Chapters 2, 10, and 12)

This patient appears to have major depression likely brought on by his wife's death. That his daughter has observed the patient to be despondent, the lack of sleep and grooming, and the apparent weight loss are all suggestive of major depression. A person can have bereavement following the loss of a loved one, but these symptoms are more consistent with major depression. Because the patient was found with a gun, has severe symptoms, and is denying illness, it is more appropriate to admit the patient to a psychiatric hospital than to arrange for outpatient treatment. Neurological consultation and nutritional therapy may be important components of this patient's management once he has been placed in a safe setting.

50. d (Chapters 2 and 10)

The suicide rate in Caucasian males over age 65 is five times that of the general population. Psychiatric disorders, especially major depression, also increase the risk of suicide. Hopelessness about the future increases the risk of suicide. Weight loss, decreased sleep, and poor grooming are associated with major depression but have not been shown to be strong indicators for increased suicide risk.

51. d (Chapters 12 and 17)

Appropriate initial therapy for this patient would include an antidepressant medication. Mirtazapine is often used in elderly individuals and improves sleep and appetite. Buspirone is sometimes used as an adjunct to antidepressant treatment but is approved for treating generalized anxiety disorder. Dialectical behavioral psychotherapy has been demonstrated to be effective mainly in the treatment of borderline personality disorder. Propanolol does not have a role as monotherapy in treating major depression and may exacerbate or cause symptoms of depression. Valproate is a mood stabilizer medication most appropriate for treating mania in bipolar disorder. This patient does not display evidence of mania.

52. b (Chapters 2 and 12)

Electroconvulsive therapy is an appropriate treatment option in an elderly individual with life-threatening depression. Decreasing the mirtazapine would not improve, but might worsen this patient's condition. Cognitive-behavioral therapy is a useful treatment for mild to moderate depression but is not appropriate given the severity of this patient's symptoms (but might be an important therapy once he improves somewhat). Multivitamins may be important for general good health but do not treat depression per se. Gabapentin is used for seizure disorders and neuropathic pain of some types but has not been demonstrated to be effective in severe depression.

53. d (Chapter 1)

Panic disorder with a panic attack might cause a disturbance in a public place but odd accusations, pressured speech, and other signs of paranoia would not be present. Heroin intoxication usually presents with a quiet, sedated condition, with decreased heart rate and respirations. Paranoia is also not usually a component of heroin intoxication. Attention-deficit/hyperactivity disorder might present with excessive motor activity but, again, paranoia, pressured speech, and agitation are not consistent with this condition. Schizophrenia, paranoid subtype, is associated with agitation, paranoia, and disheveled appearance. Therefore, this is the best diagnostic choice among the provided options. Hypothyroidism generally presents with apathy, depression, psychomotor retardation if severe. Hyperthyroidism might mimic some of the patient's symptoms, such as pressured speech or agitation. Of note, there is not sufficient evidence provided in this vignette to make a formal diagnosis of schizophrenia. The time course of the patient's illness, reversible medical causes, drug-induced paranoia, and other psychiatric conditions (such as schizoaffective disorder, mania with psychosis, or depression with psychosis) should all be carefully considered.

54. d (Chapters 9 and 15)

The clinical history is most consistent with a diagnosis of narcolepsy, a condition characterized by daytime sleep attacks, cataplexy (sudden, reversible, bilateral loss of skeletal muscle tone), sleep paralysis (temporary paralysis upon awakening from sleep), and REM sleep intrusions (experienced as sudden vivid dreams that may intrude into the waking state. If experienced at sleep onset, the REM intrusions are called hypnagogic hallucinations. If experienced at awakening, the REM intrusions are called hypnopompic hallucinations.) Modafinil is an approved treatment for narcolepsy and enhances daytime alertness. Continuous positive airway pressure at night to improve abnormal breathing is an appropriate treatment for breathing-related sleep disorder. Administration of Ambien at bedtime is an appropriate short-term treatment for insomnia. Valproic acid is used in the treatment of bipolar disorder and seizure disorder but not for narcolepsy. The patient's drop attacks with retained consciousness do not suggest a diagnosis of seizure disorder. Sleepiness in the absence of mood symptoms does not suggest a diagnosis of bipolar disorder. Olanzapine, an atypical antipsychotic medication, is quite sedating and would likely exacerbate daytime sleepiness.

55. c (Chapters 5 and 8)

Relatively acute onset agitation and confusion in the intensive care unit setting is commonly due to delirium. A psychotic disorder can be associated with agitation, but no history of psychotic symptoms is provided. Dementia is a risk factor for the development of delirium, but the onset of dementia is usually quite gradual, is not part of the patient's prior history, and would be uncommon in this age group. Antisocial personality disorder is associated with traits that might include agitation or threatening behavior but antisocial personality disorder is not directly associated with confusion. Akathisia resulting from medication administration, especially administration of typical antipsychotics (neuroleptics), is a common cause of agitation but not confusion in the intensive care unit setting. Opiates and antibiotics are not likely to produce akathisia.

56. d (Chapters 5 and 8)

An all-too-common cause of delirium in the intensive care unit setting, especially following traumatic injury, is the presence of alcohol withdrawal delirium potentially complicated by Wernicke's encephalopathy. The elevations in liver enzymes coupled with a relative pancytopenia and a history of liver problems is consistent with a diagnosis of alcohol dependence although other medical causes of these findings should be ruled out. Administration of intravenous thiamine is a critical treatment to prevent the development of irreversible brain damage as seen in Wernicke's encephalopathy.

57. d (Chapter 5)

At this point, the primary diagnostic consideration is alcohol withdrawal delirium. Alcohol withdrawal delirium is a life-threatening complication of untreated alcohol withdrawal that typically starts 48 to 72 hours after abrupt cessation of alcohol intake in alcohol-dependent individuals. The patient has elevated heart rate, blood pressure, and body temperature—symptoms consistent with autonomic hyperarousal. The treatment of choice is a benzodiazepine medication to prevent further deterioration and prevent seizure. Buspirone is a medication approved for generalized anxiety but does not treat autonomic hyperarousal. Propanolol alone or clonidine alone might reduce aspects of sympathetic activation but would actually mask the severity of the withdrawal and would not help to prevent seizure. Intravenous hydration, along with supplementation of magnesium, folate, and thiamine, is often an important supportive treatment in alcohol withdrawal but does not treat the life-threatening symptom of seizure and autonomic hyperarousal.

58. e (Chapter 5)

Naltrexone is an opiate antagonist medication that is approved for use in alcohol dependence. Naltrexone does not treat alcohol withdrawal, but helps reduce alcohol intake. Naltrexone as a pharmacological treatment should be confined with psychosocial treatments such as attendance at Alcoholics Anonymous and participation in psychotherapy. Naltrexone should not be used in patients who continue to take opiate pain relievers because the medication will precipitate acute opiate withdrawal. Benzodiazepine medications are indicated in the treatment of alcohol withdrawal but have a high risk of abuse and are generally not indicated for post-detoxification treatment. Antidepressant medications may be important adjunct therapy in individuals who have depression that persists after alcohol detoxification but are not generally indicated for treating alcohol abuse or dependence. An antihypertensive medication might be appropriate if a patient has persistently elevated blood pressure following alcohol detoxification, but many individuals in acute alcohol withdrawal have markedly elevated blood pressure that normalizes following detoxification. An opiate analgesic medication is not indicated because the patient has already been tapered from opiate analgesics, suggesting that he no longer requires opiates for acute pain relief.

59. a (Chapter 7)

This patient exhibits the common features of a person with a developmental disability. The social difficulties and getting lost in small details while missing the big picture are common manifestations of either autism or Asperger's disorder. The main distinguishing feature is the presence or absence of language difficulties. In Asperger's disorder, language function is preserved, whereas in autism language is often severely impaired. Asperger's disorder tends to be diagnosed later than autism and IQ is largely preserved in Asperger's disorder but often impaired in autism. Although patients with Asperger's disorder may appear to avoid social contact, this is secondary to the recurrent experiences of social rejection that are common for children with Asperger's disorder. Anxiety should always be ruled out, as should posttraumatic stress disorder. Children with either condition can be quite withdrawn and awkward socially.

60. e (Chapter 18)

The three elements commonly recognized in Informed Consent include information, capacity, and consent. Information is the content of the proposed treatment and the alternatives to treatment, including potential effects of failing to treat. Capacity requires that a person possess the ability to understand, appreciate, reason, and express a choice. This patient has expressed a choice. Consent must be given voluntarily, namely, must not involve subtle or overt coercion.

61. a (Chapter 18)

The *Tarasoff* decisions held that therapists have a reasonable duty to warn potential victims of threats made by patients in treatment. Although there are many different legal interpretations of this decision (also called the duty to warn or protect), it is important for practicing physicians to know the rules in their jurisdiction. The M'Naghten rule refers to the insanity defense. *Griswold v. Connecticut* is not pertinent. The duty to warn is based on initial rulings by the California Supreme Court and is not based on Swedish Common Law. Negligence is an element of medical malpractice.

62. c (Chapter 5)

The patient's symptom complex is consistent with that of intoxication with psychostimulant drugs such as cocaine. The patient likely has myocardial ischemia caused by cocaine-induced coronary artery vasospasm. The patient is at risk for myocardial infarction, cardiac arrhythmia, or stroke. In a patient who presents with this symptom complex, it is most important to treat the patient as any other patient with an acute myocardial infarction or acute myocardial ischemia depending on the electrocardiogram and other findings. However, ruling out drugs of abuse as a cause of this event is critical to future treatment and monitoring of this patient. An abdominal ultrasound is not likely to be of use unless the patient complains of abdominal pain or other signs suggesting splenic infarction or abdominal aneurysm rupture. An electroencephalogram is unlikely to be of use in an alert patient who has no evidence of altered mental status or headache. Hematocrit will not aid in the immediate diagnosis of the patient's condition. Liver function tests might be of use in such a patient if there are risk factors for alcoholic hepatitis or viral hepatitis, but they are not critical to the current diagnosis.

63. d (Chapter 5)

At present, the only diagnosis that can be made with confidence is that of myocardial infarction. The patient quite likely has cocaine abuse or cocaine dependence. However, to make a diagnosis of cocaine dependence, one would need to know that the patient had at least three symptoms consistent with tolerance, withdrawal, repeated unintended excessive use, persistent failed efforts to cut down, excessive time spent trying to obtain the substance, cocaine-related reductions in social, occupational, or recreational activities, and continued use despite awareness that cocaine is causing psychological or physical difficulties. Since this patient presented on multiple occasions to the emergency ward with chest pain following cocaine use, he is probably aware of the association between use of the drug and chest pain, and would therefore meet the last criterion (awareness of physical difficulties). We do not yet have evidence for the other criteria. Polydrug abuse or at least polydrug exposure might also be found in this patient but the current evidence does not yet support that diagnosis. Antisocial personality disorder requires a consistent and sustained pattern of disregard for social rules. This patient may have engaged in illegal activity but this is common among cocaine users in the absence of antisocial personality disorder. Malingering is diagnosed when a person deceives to obtain secondary gain. Denial of drug use is remarkably common among drug-addicted or drug-abusing individuals and is not necessarily a symptom of malingering.

64. b (Chapters 5 and 8)

Alcohol-induced persistent amnestic disorder (Korsakoff's psychosis) is associated with damage to the hippocampus, fornix, and mammillary bodies. Damage to these structures is thought to be caused by thiamine deficiency. The brainstem and frontal lobes, thalamus and cingulate gyrus, caudate and putamen, and cerebellum are not brain regions associated with amnestic disorder in alcoholism.

65. e (Chapters 3 and 14)

The patient has the classic symptoms of panic disorder. Anxiety disorders have been most strongly associated with alterations in the inhibitory neurotransmitter GABA. Serotonin and norepinephrine are also implicated in the pathophysiology of these conditions. Glycine is associated with inhibitory transmission in the spinal cord. Melatonin is associated with sleep disturbances. Substance P and enkephalin are most notably associated with pain.

66. d (Chapter 17)

The boy is struggling with Erikson's life cycle known as industry versus inferiority. Between the ages of 5 and 13 children struggle with developing a sense of self based on the things that they create. Caregivers provide for a sense of mastery by teaching and giving feedback. In this case, the child is struggling with what his performance on the soccer field implies about his general worthiness. The father is teaching and guiding his son in the sport, which is undoubtedly promoting the son's psychological development. Intimacy versus isolation, answer a, occurs later in development in young adulthood. Identity versus role confusion occurs just after identity versus inferiority and corresponds to adolescence. Initiative versus guilt precedes identity versus inferiority at ages 3 to 5 and involves the feelings of guilt that ensue when a child first has enough autonomy to explore the world including things that the parents may find disturbing. Finally, ego integrity versus despair involves late life acceptance of one's place in the life cycle versus regret of unfulfilled earlier life desires.

67. a (Chapter 9)

The patient holds a perception that her nose is crooked and, therefore, ugly that does not appear to be true. This is body dysmorphic disorder. She is extremely preoccupied with this perceived problem with her physical appearance to the point where she has sought surgical remediation. The patient does not gain satisfaction from showing her body to others as in exhibitionism. Although many clinicians may find themselves feeling annoyed with her preoccupation, she does not have the other clinically troubling features of a person with borderline personality disorder. She does feel scrutinized in public places, which suggests social phobia but her feelings are only in relation to her perception that her nose is crooked. Finally, people with posttraumatic stress disorder have anxiety and present in emergency rooms with nonspecific distress but do not have a pre-occupation with a particular part of their body.

68. b (Chapter 8)

Although there can be large amount of overlap of symptoms between Alzheimer's disease, Pick's disease, and vascular dementia, Pick's disease is generally characterized by an onset of personality change and a decline in function at work and home.

Imaging studies and presentation help make the diagnosis. At autopsy the differences are readily apparent on pathologic review. Pick's disease is marked by "Pick bodies" and neurons have a ballooned appearance. This is not seen in Alzheimer's disease, which is characterized by the plaques and tangles. Vascular dementia is more commonly characterized by either multiple cortical infarcts; subcortical small vessel disease, or strategically placed infarcts. Pick's disease is also typically restricted to the frontal and anterior temporal lobes. Huntington's chorea generally presents with a movement disorder followed by emotional lability or depression and then dementia. Creutzfeldt–Jakob's disease presents with the clinical triad of myoclonus, dementia and abnormal electroencephalogram. Spongiform encephalopathy is present at autopsy.

69. b (Chapter 17)

The patient was likely undergoing some kind of psychoanalytic psychotherapy. The focus on early childhood and the multiple sessions per week are common features of this type of therapy. The focus on relationships indicates that the therapist may have been using object-relations theory, a common form of psychoanalysis, to guide the treatment. If it were cognitive-behavioral therapy, the focus would have been on more present-day thoughts and their impact on feelings. Interpersonal therapy is a short-term therapy that focuses on specific aspects of present-day relationships. Behavior therapy uses behavioral principles of reinforcement and aversion to effect specific behavioral changes (e.g., losing weight, quitting smoking). Finally, dialectical behavior therapy is another therapy that focuses on present-day thoughts and feelings to help patients with borderline personality disorder to manage intolerable feelings and decrease self-destructive behaviors.

70. d (Chapter 15)

The medication is probably naltrexone. Naltrexone has been shown to decrease frequency and intensity of alcoholic relapse. It also does not cause illness when alcohol is consumed with it as does disulfiram (Antabuse). Zolpidem is a non-benzodiazepine sleep aid, buspirone is a non-benzodiazepine anxiolytic, and metoclopramide is a medication that is approved for gastroesophageal reflux disease and is also used off-label for migraines.

71. a (Chapter 14)

Lorazepam, oxazepam, and temazepam are benzodiazepines metabolized primarily by conjugation and do not have active metabolizes. Clonazepam is a long-acting benzodiazepine but does not have long-acting metabolites. Diazepam and chlordiazepoxide are metabolized mainly by glucuronidation and have long-acting metabolites. Thus, these two medications are prone to accumulate in individuals with impaired hepatic metabolism and may cause benzodiazepine toxicity. Buspirone is not a benzodiazepine and is not used for alcohol detoxification.

72. b (Chapter 8)

The patient has multiple risk factors for vascular-related dementia, including cigarette smoking, hypercholesterolemia, hypertension, type 2 diabetes mellitus, and coronary artery disease. Patients with these risk factors often show nonspecific brain white matter disease on MRI and should have slowed progression of dementia if treated for the underlying risk factors. Huntington's disease is an autosomal dominant inheritance; Creutzfeldt–Jacob is prion-linked; Parkinson's disease is due to degeneration in monoamine and other brain neurons; HIV is associated with exposure to the HIV virus.

73. b (Chapter 9)

The sexual response cycle is divided into four stages: Desire—Initial stage of sexual response; consists of sexual fantasies and the urge to have sex. Excitement—Consists of physiologic arousal and feeling of sexual pleasure. Orgasm—Peaking sexual pleasure; usually associated with ejaculation in males. Resolution—Physiologic relaxation associated with a sense of well-being. In males, there is usually a refractory period for further excitement and orgasm. Plateau is not a phase of the sexual response cycle.

74. e (Chapter 9)

Breathing-related sleep disorder is a condition characterized by disordered breathing during sleep that results in frequent awakening and fragmentation of nighttime sleep with resultant daytime sleepiness. The patient's syndrome complex is consistent with sleep apnea syndrome, a type of breathing-related sleep dysfunction consisting of recurrent episodes of apnea while sleeping. The presence of loud snoring and choking or gasping during sleep is a cardinal sign of this condition.

75. d (Chapter 5)

Barbiturate withdrawal can be fairly dangerous and can include hyperpyrexia, seizure, and potentially death. Withdrawal from crack cocaine, crystal methamphetamine, and marijuana is generally self-limited. Occasionally, the patient can appear psychotic during intoxication with these agents. Withdrawal from crack cocaine and crystal methamphetamine is generally characterized by fatigue, depression, nightmares, headache, sweating, muscle cramps, and hunger. Nicotine withdrawal is characterized by irritability, fatigue, insomnia, and difficulty concentrating.

ANSWERS

Bibliography

Andreasen NC, Black DW. *Introductory textbook of psychiatry*. 3rd ed. Washington, DC: American Psychiatric Publishing, 2001.

Baldessarini RJ. *Chemotherapy in psychiatry: Principles and practice*. Cambridge, Mass: Harvard University Press, 1985.

Corsini RJ, Wedding D. *Current psychotherapies*. 6th ed. Belmont, Calif: Wadsworth, 2000.

Davison GC, Neale JM, Kring AM. *Abnormal psychology*. 9th ed. New York: John Wiley & Sons, 2003.

Diagnostic and statistical manual of mental disorders. 4th ed, text rev. Washington, DC: American Psychiatric Association, 2000.

Hales RE, Yudofsky SC. *Textbook of clinical psychiatry*. 4th ed. Washington, DC: American Psychiatric Publishing, 2003.

Physicians' desk reference. 59th ed. Montvale, NJ: Medical Economics, 2005.

Ropper AH, Brown RH. *Adams and Victor's principles of neurology*. 8th ed. New York: McGraw-Hill Professional, 2005.

Rosenbaum JF, Arana GW, Hyman SE, et al. *Handbook of psychiatric drug therapy*. 5th ed. Philadelphia: Lippincott Williams & Wilkins, 2005.

Sadock BJ, Sadock VA, Kaplan HI. *Comprehensive textbook of psychiatry*. 8th ed. Philadelphia: Lippincott Williams & Wilkins, 2004.

Index

Page numbers followed by italic *f* or *t* refer to illustrations or tables, respectively.